Bovine Practice

The *In Practice* Handbooks Series

Series Editor: Edward Boden

Past and present members of *In Practice* Editorial Board

Professor J. Armour, Chairman 1979–1989,
Dean, Veterinary Faculty, University of Glasgow

Titles in print:
Feline Practice
Canine Practice
Equine Practice
Bovine Practice
Sheep and Goat Practice
Swine Practice

The *In Practice* Handbooks

Bovine Practice

Edited by E. Boden
Executive Editor, *In Practice*

Baillière Tindall

LONDON   PHILADELPHIA   TORONTO   SYDNEY   TOKYO

Baillière Tindall   24–28 Oval Road
W. B. Saunders   London NW1 7DX

The Curtis Center
Independence Square West
Philadelphia, PA 19106–3399, USA

55 Horner Avenue
Toronto, Ontario, M8Z 4X6, Canada

Harcourt Brace Jovanovich Group
(Australia) Pty Ltd
30–52 Smidmore Street
Marrickville
NSW 2204, Australia

Harcourt Brace Jovanovich Japan Inc
Ichibancho Central Building
22–1 Ichibancho
Chiyoda-ku, Tokyo 102, Japan

Typeset by Photo-graphics, Honiton, Devon
Printed and bound in Hong Kong by Dah Hua Printing Press Co., Ltd.

A catalogue record for this book is available from
the British Library

ISBN 0–7020–1556–3

Contents

Fertility

Disease and Medical Problems

BVD virus and other pathogens. Mucosal disease.
Differential diagnosis. Laboratory techniques for
diagnosis of BVD virus. Deer and sheep.
Conclusions

Control

Contributors

A. Andrews, Department of Veterinary Medicine and Animal Husbandry, Royal Veterinary College, North Mymms, Hatfield, Herts, UK

I. Baker, 49 Cambridge Street, Aylesbury, Bucks, UK

P. Ball, High Park, Wootton Courtenay, Minehead, Somerset, UK

J. Brownlie, Immunopathology Division, AFRC Institute for Animal Health, Compton, Newbury, Berks, UK

B. Drew, Ministry of Agriculture, Fisheries and Food, Coley Park, Reading, Berks, UK

R. G. Hemingway, Department of Veterinary Animal Husbandry, University of Glasgow, Glasgow, UK

J. E. Hillerton, Milking and Mastitis Centre, AFRC Institute for Animal Health, Compton, Berks, UK

T. O. Jones, Ministry of Agriculture, Fisheries and Food, Veterinary Investigation Centre, Sutton Bonnington, Leicester, UK

J. Kelly, Department of Veterinary Clinical Studies, University of Edinburgh, and Royal (Dick) School of Veterinary Studies, Easter Bush, Nr Roslin, Midlothian, UK

B. Lowman, The Scottish Agricultural College, Animal Sciences Division, Bush Estate, Penicuik, UK

D. Noakes, Department of Large Animal Medicine, Royal Veterinary College, North Mymms, Hatfield, Herts, UK

L. Petrie, Department of Veterinary Medicine, University of Saskatchewan, Saskatoon, Canada

J. Pinsent, Saxon Place, Langford, Bristol, Avon, UK

R. Plenderleith, Legbourne House, Legbourne, Lincs, UK

D. Snodgrass, Division of Microbiology, Animal Diseases Research Association, Moredun Institute, Edinburgh, UK

M. Vaughan, Veterinary Surgeon, Westmoor Veterinary Clinic, Tavistock, Devon, UK

A. J. Webster, Department of Animal Husbandry, Bristol University Veterinary School, Bristol, UK

D. White, Lecturer in Veterinary Medicine, Department of Veterinary Medicine, Royal Veterinary College, North Mymms, Hatfield, Herts, UK

Foreword

In Practice was started in 1979 as a clinical supplement to *The Veterinary Record*. Its carefully chosen, highly illustrated articles specially commissioned from leaders in their field were aimed specifically at the practitioner. They have proved extremely popular with experienced veterinarians and students alike. The editorial board, chaired for the first 10 years by Professor James Armour, was particularly concerned to emphasize differential diagnosis.

In response to consistent demand, articles from *In Practice*, updated and revised by the authors, are now published in convenient handbook form. Each book deals with a particular species or group of related animals.

E. Boden

Production

CHAPTER 1

Health and Welfare of Animals in Modern Husbandry Systems – Dairy Cattle

A. JOHN WEBSTER

INTRODUCTION

The codes of recommendations for the welfare of livestock in the UK, as drawn up by the Farm Animal Welfare Council, recognize certain basic needs (see Table 1). The welfare of animals in any husbandry system, old or new, intensive or extensive, may be evaluated in the context of these needs.

Table 1.1 Basic needs of livestock, as assessed by the Farm Animal Welfare Council.

Freedom from thirst, hunger or malnutrition – achieved by readily accessible fresh water and a diet to maintain full health and vigour

Appropriate comfort and shelter

Freedom from injury or disease – achieved by prevention or rapid diagnosis and treatment

Freedom of movement and the opportunity to express most normal patterns of behaviour

Freedom from fear

No system is perfect and these disparate needs may sometimes conflict. For example, increased freedom of movement
in young cattle *may* increase the incidence of enteritis, the
more comfortable cubicle *may* also predispose to a greater
incidence of mastitis. Conclusions as to the acceptability of a
particular system are value judgements and thus expressions
of personal opinion. However, this author believes that it is
possible to achieve a balanced judgement only if all five of the
criteria for welfare ("the five freedoms") listed are considered in
terms of the scientific understanding of the physiology, health
and behaviour of the species in question; in this case, cattle.

It is further believed that the right to good health and vigour
is the most important of the five freedoms. This inevitably
implies that less importance is attached to freedom of behavioural expression. This is perhaps an unfashionable opinion
but one which is particularly necessary when evaluating the
welfare of the dairy cow. Relative to many farm animals the
dairy cow has considerable behavioural freedom and this has
led to claims that "there are no major welfare problems in the
dairy sector" (Wilson, 1979). The more complete evaluation,
which equates welfare with good husbandry, would merit
several books. In the space available, the present article can
do no more than highlight some major problems and suggest
a few possible solutions.

CALF REARING

The natural circumstances for a calf are, of course, to be born
on range or at pasture and to run with its mother. The beef
cow on open range makes a pretty good job of rearing its own
offspring, provided that the cow itself is well nourished and
in a healthy environment. The calf born to the dairy cow,
however, is routinely submitted to more insults to normal
development than any other farm animal. It is taken from its
mother shortly after birth, deprived of its natural food, whole
cow's milk, and fed one of a variety of cheaper liquid
substitutes. Even these are deemed unduly expensive and
the rearer is under pressure to wean calves on to solid,
carbohydrate-based foods as soon as possible. Furthermore,
intensive calf-rearing units usually take in calves after passage

through two or more markets. Problems of markets are outside the scope of this article but it is fair to say that they do not make things any easier for the calf or the stockman. The options for rearing calves from the dairy herd are listed in Table 1.2.

BEHAVIOUR

Rearing calves for veal in individual crates has come under intense criticism, mostly for suppression of behaviour. A research team from the University of Bristol, in association with the State veterinary service, recently looked in detail at the development of behaviour and the incidence of injury and disease in calves on 72 veal units incorporating all the major rearing systems. The behaviour of suckler calves at pasture with their mothers was used as a standard against which to assess the others.

The spontaneous maintenance behaviour of early-weaned calves and veal calves raised in groups was, in general, very similar to that of suckled calves at pasture. Veal calves raised in individual crates without solid food showed several abnormalities of behaviour. At 2 weeks of age they remained standing for abnormally long periods. They seemed to be insecure on the wooden slats and reluctant to change position. Above 10 weeks of age they were too big to adopt a normal sleeping position in crates only 750 mm wide. Denied normal social contact and access to dry food they spent abnormally long periods in purposeless oral activity such as licking the walls of their cages. Paradoxically, therefore, the veal calf

Table 1.2 Options for rearing calves from dairy herds.

Bucket feeding once or twice per day in individual pens to weaning at 5–6 weeks

Group rearing with unrestricted access to milk replacer via teat feeders to weaning at 5–6 weeks

Rearing for veal in individual crates on liquid feed from buckets with no access to roughage or other dry food

Rearing for veal in groups in straw yards with unrestricted access to liquid feed via teats isolated in a crate may spend less time at rest than one reared in a group and given freedom to exercise and play.

The response of calves to the presence of man or any other departure from the normal routine of the day is governed by a fine balance between curiosity and timidity. Figures 1.1 and 1.2 illustrate the response of calves to a complete novelty (balloons) in the familiar environment of their own pen and shortly after being moved into a strange yard. Note the position of the feet. In Fig. 1.1 curiosity is all and the calf approaches the balloon with confidence. Outside the familiar environment (Fig. 1.2) the curiosity is still there but the calf is braced for flight.

Most calves accustomed to the presence of man and the sights and sounds of normal farm activity display little, if any, evidence of fear. Veal calves reared in individual crates in enclosed, darkened buildings which receive very little in the way of extraneous stimuli, are, for the most part, very quiet. However, sudden movements can severely startle one or two calves and the noise created by them in wooden crates causes the panic to spread.

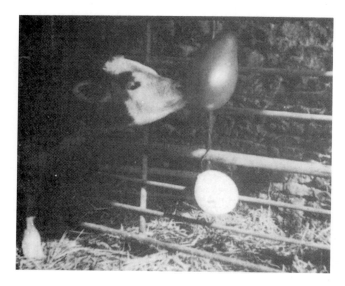

Fig. 1.1
Investigation by calves of a novel object in a familiar environment.

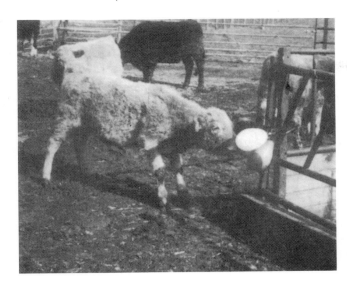

Fig. 1.2
Investigation of a
novel object in a
strange environment.

INFECTIOUS DISEASE

The main reason advocated for keeping any calf in an individual pen for the first weeks of life has been to restrict the spread of infectious disease. When group-rearing systems with dispensers, which give calves unrestricted access to milk replacer via teats, were first introduced in the late 1950s, this fear appeared to be well founded. More recently, however, improvements in the quality of milk replacers and means for their delivery have made group rearing a much more attractive prospect.

Work conducted at Bristol by Webster *et al.* (1985a,b) (see Table 1.3) found that the number of bought-in calves requiring treatment for infectious disease was about three times greater than for home-reared calves. The incidence of enteric and respiratory disease on affected farms (i.e. those that did not escape disease altogether) revealed that the spread of enteric infection was certainly no worse when calves were fed from teats and were reared in groups than when they were bucket fed in individual pens. Indeed, the findings suggest that the beneficial effects of natural feed methods fully compensate for any possible risks consequent upon direct contact between calves reared in groups. Furthermore, it was found that calves reared in groups before weaning and kept in the same groups (and often the same building) thereafter were less likely to contract respiratory disease between 6 and 14 weeks of age. The increased incidence of respiratory disease in bought-in calves before weaning at 6 weeks probably reflects a response to infection contracted in markets.

HEALTH AND PRODUCTION

A further study at Bristol (see Table 1.4) has been exploring ways of rearing veal calves in such a way as to avoid the worst insults associated with the conventional crated system yet ensure optimal health and productivity. The study involved Friesian bulls and Hereford cross Friesian heifer calves and, although the number of animals involved was relatively small, the study has generated several conclusions which are significant, not only in a statistical sense but also in terms of commercial calf husbandry and welfare.

Table 1.3 Incidence (%) of calves requiring treatment for enteric and respiratory disease on affected farms (for further details, see Webster *et al.*, 1985a,b).

	Home-reared calves		Bought-in calves
	Individual pens and buckets	Group rearing with teats	Individual pens and buckets
Percentage of all calves receiving treatment			
2–6 weeks		16	48
6–14 weeks		13	7
Treatments on affected farms Enteric disease (%)			
0–6 weeks	20	10	40
6–14 weeks	nil	nil	nil
Respiratory disease (%)			
0–6 weeks	10	10	45
6–14 weeks	40	10	15

Veal calves in crates, given access to solid food containing digestible fibre, were less subject to bouts of indigestion and inappetence. The best calves given milk only did as well as those getting 10 % dry food. The mean improvement in liveweight gain and food conversion in calves getting dry food was due to fewer "poor doers".

Calves reared in groups and bucket fed twice daily were not a success. As with early-weaned calves, the two procedures do not seem to be compatible. Abnormalities of oral behaviour such as prepuce sucking and urine drinking were also most marked in this group.

Rearing veal calves in groups with free access to milk from teats (the "Quantock" system) undoubtedly gives satisfactory standards of comfort and behavioural freedom. However, health appears to be no better than for calves in crates. Food conversion efficiency, and thus the cost of milk powder, is far worse.

The most successful approach to the rearing of veal calves is a system devised at Bristol using a computer-controlled dispenser to provide milk and solids to calves in controlled quantities. The food conversion ratio using this system was

Table 1.4 Effect of rearing system on the performance and health of veal calves at the University of Bristol.

	Crated calves		Group reared		
	Milk only	Milk + solids	Buckets	Teats *ad libitum*	Teats, milk + solids, controlled
Liveweight gain (kg/day)					
Friesian male	1.10	1.22	1.15	1.22	–
H × F female*	–	–	–	1.02	1.22
Intake (kg milk powder)					
Friesian male	202	196	200	247	–
H × F female	–	–	–	213	178
Powder:gain	1.59	1.40	1.41	1.70	1.42
Deaths and culls (%)	——— 8.8 ———		20	8.0	nil
Enteric disease (%)	——— 36 ———		33	32	6
Respiratory disease (%)	——— 8.8 ———		12	25	nil

*H × F Hereford cross Friesian

as good as for the best calves in crates. Moreover, the incidence of death and disease in these bought-in calves has been reduced to an absolute minimum. The welfare advantages are obvious.

The economic advantages of good health, coupled with food conversion efficiency, make this the system that yields the greatest gross profit margin. The feeding system is expensive (although could be made cheaper) but less expensive than costs incurred in constructing specialist buildings and equipment for rearing veal calves in crates.

DAIRY CATTLE

METABOLIC STRESS – THE OVERWORKED COW

The modern dairy cow is like a highly tuned racing car designed to run as fast as possible on very high grade fuel. As with Grand Prix cars, the results are, at best, spectacular but at least unreliable and at worst catastrophic. The amount of work done by the cow in peak lactation is immense. To achieve a comparably high work rate a human would have to jog for about 6 h a day, every day.

The metabolic problems posed by the work of lactation and some of their consequences for the welfare of the dairy cow are illustrated in Fig. 1.3. To achieve in early lactation a milk yield of 35 l/day the work done by the mammary gland and other organs, such as the liver, which make substrates available to the mammary gland, greatly exceeds the amount of energy-yielding nutrients that the cow can consume from a properly balanced diet. The animal must therefore mobilize energy from its own body reserves, chiefly fat. Up to a point this is normal and healthy. However, excessive fat mobilization leads to accumulation of ketone bodies (ketosis or acetonaemia) and, in many cases, to fatty infiltration of the cells of the liver. The cow then loses its appetite which makes matters worse. Humans with ketosis and liver damage feel extremely unwell and it would be reasonable to assume the same for cows.

The food intake of a cow is determined in part by its metabolic needs (i.e. a high-yielding cow is hungrier than a dry one) but is also constrained by the limits of gut fill.

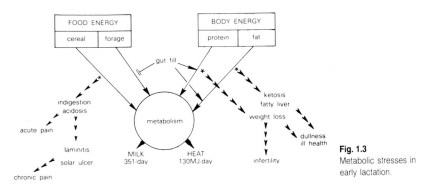

Fig. 1.3
Metabolic stresses in
early lactation.

Forages such as hay and silage are fermented relatively slowly
and a cow will eat these to its capacity long before meeting
its metabolic needs. All feeding systems for cattle increase the
ratio of concentrate (cereal based) to forage feeds at the onset
of lactation. Once again, this is normal and healthy, up to a
point. Excess intake of rapidly fermented concentrated feeds
leads to indigestion, ruminal acidosis and the disruption of
the normal rumen microflora. This provokes, at least, acute
discomfort and loss of production. In more severe cases the
primary ruminal upset can lead to metabolic acidosis and
inflammation of the sensitive laminae of the feet. In its acute
form this causes the cow severe and enduring pain. It can
also lead to separation of the sensitive and horny laminae,
rotation of the hoof and a predisposition to subsequent
ulceration of the sole.

COMFORT AND CUBICLE DESIGN

The dairy cow lies down to rest for about 10 h every day.
Ideally, it requires a comfortable, hygienic area which it can
approach without disturbance, wherein it can stand up and
lie down without difficulty and where it can rest in comfort
and security, but in social contact with other cows.

At their best, spacious yards generously bedded down with
clean straw provide ideal standards for both comfort and
surface hygiene. To be effective, this system requires about
1 t of straw per cow per year, which is only economically
viable on farms which make their own straw. For the majority

of dairy cows the current question is what constitutes the ideal cubicle.

Cubical dimensions

The dimensions should be sufficient to accommodate the largest cows in the herd. The cow should be able to stand in comfort with all four feet in the cubicle but urinate and defecate in the passage. Since the animal almost invariably does these activities while standing up, this can be controlled in a cubicle of any size by judicious placing of the headrail or brisket board. The cow also needs space to lunge forwards as it stands up and lies down. The recommended dimensions for a 600–700 kg Friesian cow are 2.3 m long by 1.2 m wide (Table 1.5) but, from the cow's point of view, a cubicle cannot be too long provided the floor is well drained and the stockman adjusts the headrails intelligently and removes any excreta from the backs of the cubicle beds twice daily. Cubicles that are too short predispose to mastitis, teat injuries and lameness.

Divisions between cubicles

The divisions between cubicles have evolved in response to experience and to fashion and there is a wide range of more or less successful designs. The objectives are to align cows properly in their own cubicle, to prevent their feet interfering with or injuring their neighbours and to minimize the risk of injury to limb or teat as the cow changes position. As a general rule, the less pipework or other rigid material by which the cow might get trapped, the better.

Table 1.5 Cubicle design for Friesian/Holstein cows (600–700 kg).

Length – 2.3 m
Width – 1.2 m
Forward lying room – 0.7–1.0 m – adjust headrail
Bed – reconcile comfort and hygiene
Slope – 70–80 mm front to back; no lateral slope

Cubicle bed

The cubicle bed should be designed to ensure comfort and hygiene. It is important to ensure a clean, dry lying area to minimize the risk of environmental mastitis, i.e. that associated with bad housing rather than faulty milking techniques and mainly caused by *Escherichia coli* or *Streptococcus uberis*. A survey of mastitis in the British dairy herd made during 1977–1978 attributed about 5 % of all cases of mastitis to infection with these organisms (Wilson and Richards, 1980). By 1982 environmental mastitis was accounting for about 35 % of all recorded cases (Wilesmith *et al.*, 1986). Clearly, modern housing (especially cubicle housing) is failing to ensure freedom from this painful disease.

The size and shape of a dairy cow are such that the pressure exerted at rest on skin and bone at sites like the carpus and tarsus (and the shear forces exerted when in motion) are far more severe than those which man would experience if lying on the same surface. The UK code of welfare for cattle states that cows should not be kept in a totally slatted area. On reflection, the Farm Animal Welfare Council has concluded that this recommendation should apply only to dairy cows. It is acceptable, although not ideal, to keep small, non-lactating beef cows on concrete slats in areas where alternatives such as straw bedding are prohibitively expensive, as in the northern isles of Scotland. It is not acceptable for beef cows with calves.

When cows are given a selection of bedding materials in cubicles there is no doubt that their choice is motivated by the desire for comfort and that, except in extremely cold environments, their first priority for comfort is a good mattress.

A cubicle bed may consist of material such as straw, woodshavings, paper or sand. All of these can provide satisfactory standards of comfort and hygiene if well managed but are dangerous if allowed to become wet and dirty. Synthetic cow beds are preferred in direct proportion to their springiness and cushioning effects and can, of course, be kept very clean.

Bare concrete and similar unyielding materials do not provide suitable beds for lactating dairy cattle. It is most unlikely that the provision of a suitable bed can ever be justified on economic grounds alone. It becomes, therefore, a criterion of good welfare that can only be ensured by legislation.

LAMENESS

Lameness, mainly that caused by painful damage to the foot, is probably the most common single cause of distress to dairy cows at this time. Surveys of cases of lameness treated by veterinary surgeons indicate an average annual incidence of about 4–6 % (Rowlands *et al.*, 1983). When cases treated by the farmer are included, the annual incidence appears to be about 25 % (Whitaker *et al.*, 1983). Foot lameness is the consequence of a number of distinct pathological conditions the most important of which are listed in Table 1.6.

The factors that predispose to lameness in dairy cows include the following:

(1) Conformation. The shape of the modern dairy cow undoubtedly predisposes to foot damage. For example, over 70 % of solar ulcers occur on the lateral claws of the hind feet.
(2) Nutrition. Most cases of laminitis and its sequelae, white line disease and solar ulcer, occur in early lactation. It has been difficult to obtain conclusive proof of the link between laminitis and high intakes of rapidly fermented starches (and possibly proteins) but the circumstantial evidence linking the two is very strong.
(3) Environment. Interdigital necrobacillosis can usually be attributed to a wound inflicted by a sharp object in filthy conditions, e.g. when cows walk through a muddy farm gate.

Table 1.6 Main causes of foot lameness in cattle.

Interdigital necrobacillosis – "Foul-in-the foot"; inflammation associated with *Fusiformis necrophorus* originating in the interdigital space

Pododermatitis – Inflammation or trauma to the sole of the foot progressing in many cases to solar ulcer

White line disease – Damage leading to separation of the junction between the wall and sole

Laminitis – Acute or chronic inflammation of the sensitive laminae of the foot

It tends to occur most frequently in cows at pasture on smaller, poorer, less productive farms. Control is simple, in theory; make the walkways cleaner and safer. In practice, however, this may be prohibitively expensive for the small farmer.

Damage to the sole of the foot, whether primary or consequent upon laminitis, is primarily a condition of housed cows. From the available evidence it is not possible to say whether one form of housing is better or worse than another, but it is almost certain that the overall problem has become worse over the last 20 years.

Although a great deal is known about the pathology and pathogenesis of foot lameness, our failure to prevent this state of affairs can reasonably be attributed to ignorance as to its aetiology. Most explanations are incomplete and most surveys stop short of asking the most interesting questions. Changes in patterns of dairy husbandry, such as cubicle housing, the switch from hay to silage and increased feeding of concentrates, have all come under attack and with some justification. However, there is as yet no coherent picture of how these and other factors interact to damage the feet. This problem continues therefore to be a high priority for research based both on laboratory studies and field work.

It is absolutely vital that the sponsors of research be made aware that a stated commitment to increase the priority for research related to farm animal welfare does not just mean a little bit more money for ethology but rather a continuous commitment to new knowledge to reduce suffering caused by painful and crippling disease.

MASTITIS

Mastitis causes not only pain to the cow (and sometimes death) but severe economic loss to the farmer. Here then the interests of economics and welfare are at one. The aetiology and control of mastitis are far too complex to consider here. However, there is evidence that the incidence is declining as farmers respond to economic incentives to improve milk hygiene. The advent of loose housing in cubicles has increased the incidence of environmental mastitis but, on the other hand, has reduced the incidence of mastitis associated with improper hygiene or technique at the time of milking. A farmer who, with the help of his veterinary surgeon, keeps the incidence of mastitis below 30 cases per 100 cows per year is probably doing as well as he can. When the incidence is higher, the problem is one that requires skilled treatment according to the conditions specific to the farm in question.

TRANSPORT AND SLAUGHTER

At the end of its life, the dairy cow becomes a red meat animal. The welfare of such animals in lairage and at the point of slaughter has been reviewed in detail by the Farm Animal Welfare Council. Here the most serious causes for concern relate to casualty and emergency slaughter.

Casualty animals are those which are not in severe pain but which are decreed to be suffering from injury or disease sufficient to require slaughter as soon as possible. Such animals may be transported to slaughterhouses. It is unrealistic to expect local abattoirs to be available for casualty slaughter 24 h a day, 7 days a week.

Emergency cases are those where the animal has experienced severe injury and cannot move or be moved without enduring severe pain. Here, the Farm Animal Welfare Council recommends that the animals be killed humanely on the spot, despite the loss of value that ensues. All this is very laudable but it faces the hard-pressed dairy farmer with an appallingly difficult ethical dilemma which may be expressed "Does my charity and compassion to one old cow extend to (say) £350?".

In this, as in other welfare problems cited earlier, it is important to be sympathetic to the needs of the farmer as well as to his animals. This requires a scheme that makes it neither prohibitively expensive nor particularly attractive financially for him to arrange for on-farm slaughter and veterinary certification of both emergency and some casualty cases. One possibility is a low-premium but compulsory insurance scheme run by an organization such as the Milk Marketing Board to compensate the farmer for such animals.

CONCLUSIONS

This paper has considered the major welfare problems facing cattle at the present time. Such "problems" may not necessarily be a cause for outrage but more a matter of importance which is incompletely understood or not fully under control. Solutions will emerge slowly from rational and judicious application of three fundamental principles which provide the foundations, not just for animal welfare, but for most of what we call civilization. These are:

(1)   The acquisition of new knowledge by research.
(2)   The dissemination of knowledge and ethics by education.
(3)   The enforcement of human principles (especially where they conflict with market forces) by legislation.

Few would quarrel with the first two of these three principles. Legislation is less popular because it implies bureaucracy and infringement of individual freedoms. Nevertheless, the successful farmer is one who operates efficiently within any given set of rules. Good farmers, whether they farm cattle, pigs, sheep or poultry, have nothing to fear from new sets of rules, created by law and fairly enforced.

ACKNOWLEDGEMENTS

I am grateful to David Welchman and the Animal Health Trust for giving me access to new, unpublished information on veal calves.

REFERENCES

Baggott, D. (1982). *Veterinary Record* Supplement. *In Practice* **4**, 133.
Farm Animal Welfare Council (1984). *Report on the Welfare of Livestock (Red Meat Animals) at the Time of Slaughter.* HMSO, London.
Ministry of Agriculture, Fisheries and Food (1983). *Codes of Recommendations for the Welfare of Livestock: Cattle.* Leaflet 701. Alnwick. MAFF Publications, Northumberland.
Rowlands, G. J., Russell, A. M. & Williams, L. A. (1983). *Veterinary Record* **113**, 441.

Webster, A. J. F. (1984). *Calf Husbandry, Health and Welfare*. Granada, London.

Webster, A. J. F., Saville, C., Church, B. M., Gnanasakthy, A. & Moss, R. (1985a). *British Veterinary Journal* **141**, 249.

Webster, A. J. F., Saville, C., Church, B. M., Gnanasakthy, A. & Moss, R. (1985b). *British Veterinary Journal* **141**, 472.

Whitaker, D. A., Kelly, J. M. & Smith, E. J. (1983). *Veterinary Record* **113**, 60.

Wilesmith, J. W., Francis, P. G. & Wilson, C. D. (1986). *Veterinary Record* **118**, 199.

Wilson, C. D. & Richards, M. S. (1980). *Veterinary Record* **406**, 431.

Wilson, P. N. (1979). *The Welfare of the Food Animals*, p. 9. Universities Federation for Animal Welfare, Potters Bar.

CHAPTER 2

Suckler Cow Management

BASIL LOWMAN

INTRODUCTION

The introduction of milk quotas in the EC in 1984 has led to a 12 % reduction in the number of dairy cows when compared with the peak of 1983. This reduction has had a major effect on calf supplies particularly in the UK where, traditionally, 65 % of all beef originated from the dairy herd (Fig. 2.1). The problem is further aggravated by the increasing proportion of Holstein blood being used in the UK dairy herd which adversely affects the suitability of dairy cross calves for beef production. Holstein cross Friesian steers have poorer killing out percentages and carcass conformation compared with purebred Friesian steers (Table 2.1). Because of their poorer conformation, Holstein cross carcasses produce a lower yield of saleable meat, a crucial factor in the profitability of meat wholesalers.

Also the much greater incidence of BSE in dairy herds has resulted in the retail trade associating beef from the dairy herd, particularly from intensive finishing systems, as "less marketable" compared with the more "natural" image of beef from the suckler herd.

Calf supplies for beef production have been further

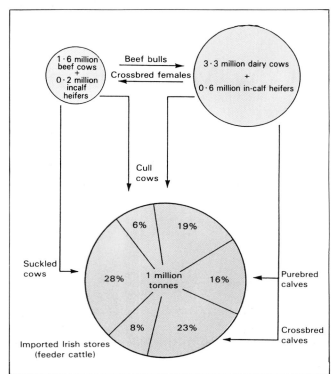

Fig. 2.1
Sources of beef in
the UK (MLC, 1978).

Table 2.1 Effect of Holstein crosses on carcass quality.

	Holstein × Friesian	Friesian
Baber *et al.* (1984)		
Carcass weight (kg)	234.5	235.9
Killing out (%)	51.2	52.1
Conformation score	2.62	3.21
% Graded	40	70
MLC (1981)		
Saleable meat (% of carcass)	70	68.5
Saleable meat in higher-priced cuts (%)	45	44

depressed with a buoyant export trade, live calf exports to mid-1987 being doubled.

As a consequence of the shortage of calves for beef production and the corresponding high prices for calves, there is renewed interest in the suckler herd. This is already being reflected in the provisional UK June census for 1987 which showed a 2.4 % increase in the number of beef cows.

EFFICIENCY AND PROFITABILITY OF SUCKLED-CALF PRODUCTION

The biological efficiency of suckled-calf production is restricted by the cow's reproductive rate (a maximum of one calf per cow per year) and an upper limit on the rate of calf liveweight gain (just over 1 kg per head per day) if slaughter weights are to be maintained with an acceptable level of carcass finish.

This biological limit to output has to cover two major fixed costs involved in keeping a beef cow. The first is the maintenance cost which, for an average beef cow, is around 18 000 MJ/year (equivalent to *c*. 9 t of average quality silage). Perhaps more important is the capital investment in the cow herself. With today's prices of over £600 for a first calved heifer, current interest charges, assuming that all the money was borrowed, would amount to almost £100 per cow per year.

As a consequence, the commercial profitability of a suckler herd is very dependent on good management. Furthermore, suckler herds can only be viable where they utilize resources on the farm which are unsuitable for other potentially more productive enterprises. Examples of this would be marginal grazing land, most noticeably the hills and uplands or, by-product feeds such as straw or vegetable waste. Perhaps, most importantly, profitable suckled-calf production can only be attained with a minimum of fixed costs in terms of machinery, buildings and labour.

The final point is the long-term nature of suckled-calf production. This is true of both the production cycle (an 18-month cycle – 9 months pregnant and 9 months of calf growth) and the lifetime performance of suckler cows. In dairying the average number of lactations per cow is three-and-a-half, resulting in an average culling age of 6 years. In comparison, suckled-calf production, to be profitable, is dependent on between six and seven calves produced per cow, resulting in an average age at culling of 9 years.

BASIC DECISIONS FOR ESTABLISHING A PROFITABLE HERD

In deciding to set up a suckler herd or reviewing an existing enterprise, there are three basic questions which should be asked:

When should the cows calve?
What breeds of cow and bull should be used?
How do I manage them?

SEASON OF CALVING

Suckler cow systems are best described by the season of calving – either spring or autumn calving. Analysis of the growth rate of calves from birth to the following autumn for four commercial herds with a 7-month calving period, beginning in October each year, are shown in Fig. 2.2.

MID-WINTER CALVING

Growth rates are severely depressed for calves born mid-winter and highlight its general unsuitability as a calving

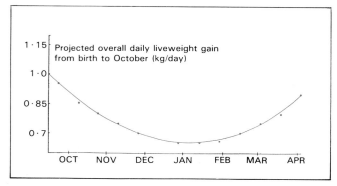

Fig. 2.2
The effect of date of birth on daily liveweight gain of calves.

period. The problems are further aggravated by mating occurring during the last few months of the winter-feeding period when cows are traditionally in their poorest condition. Wright *et al.* (1987) clearly demonstrated the problem with an average interval of 94 days between calving and the start of oestrus activity with November/December calving cows. Yet to achieve a 12-month calving interval the period from calving to conception has to be no longer than 80 days. Even cows calving in good condition (condition score 2.8 at calving) and well fed during lactation (111 MJ metabolizable energy/day) only achieved a post-partum anoestrus period of 78 days (Table 2.2).

AUTUMN CALVING

The main systems of suckled-calf production are therefore based on spring or autumn calving. Autumn calving starts no earlier than mid-August and is completed by mid-November. The exact starting date will depend on many factors, such as when the herd needs to be housed and the availability of labour to supervise calving adequately.

Traditionally autumn-calving cows suckle their calves over the summer, weaning occurring approximately 1 month before calving. Recent developments in autumn-calving herds have reduced the length of lactation by weaning calves at turnout to enable differing qualities of grassland to be grazed more efficiently. This system allows the dry, pregnant cow to be

Table 2.2 Length of post-partum anoestrus period in November/December calving cows (days).

	Condition score at calving	
	Thin (2.1)	Fit (2.8)
Feed level low (56 MJ/day)	116 (50 %)*	85 (9 %)
Feed level high (111 MJ/day)	92 (16 %)	78 (0 %)

*Figures in brackets show proportion of cows which had not started cycling at turnout.

grazed on poor-quality roughages and reduces the requirement for good-quality grazing to that required for the weaned calves. The system is particularly applicable to farms with large areas of poor-quality grazing which would be insufficient to produce good calf growth rates and, perhaps more importantly, allow the pregnant cow to regain sufficient condition. Experience suggests that approximately half an acre (0.2 hectare) of good-quality grazing can be saved for each cow weaned at turnout, compared with the traditional method of weaning in July.

SPRING CALVING

For spring-calving herds there are two distinct systems depending on when calves are sold.

Traditional

The traditional spring-calving system was based on selling weaned calves at around 6 months old in the autumn suckled-calf sales. In order to achieve reasonable calf sale weights of around 250 kg, calving occurs in late winter, normally starting towards the end of February. The exact start of calving will depend on the expected date of turnout of the herd to adequate supplies of spring grass. The objective is to start mating 1–2 weeks after turnout when cows are gaining condition rapidly and it is this which will determine the exact date of calving.

Alternative

The alternative system, often called May or June calving, has been developed where calves can be overwintered for sale the following spring, when prices per kilogram are normally above those obtained in the autumn suckled-calf sales. In this system, calving starts once the cows have been on spring grass for 1–2 weeks to minimize the risk of scour in newborn calves, a major problem with the traditional spring-calving system. Date of weaning in May calving herds is extremely flexible, ranging from late autumn, where winter housing requires cows and calves to be housed separately, through to immediately before sale in late March where ample supplies of winter feed are available for the cow.

BREED OF SUCKLER COW

Choosing the correct breed of suckler cow for the environment in which she will live is a fundamental decision influencing the long-term profitability of the enterprise. The important characteristics of a suckler cow are described below.

FERTILITY

Fertility is the single most important factor influencing the profitability of suckled-calf production. Selecting for high levels of fertility by pedigree breeding shows little, if any, response. Fertility can, however, be significantly improved by heterosis. This effect can be clearly seen from large-scale American trials where three breeds (Aberdeen Angus, Hereford and Shorthorn), similar in mature size were run in 100 cow herds and bred either purebred, purebred cows mated to a different breed of bull (two-way cross calves) or crossbred cows mated to a third breed of bull (three-way cross calves). An 8 % increase in herd output (total weight of calf weaned per 100 cows put to the bull) was gained from producing a two-way cross. A major 23 % increase in output was achieved by producing a three-way cross calf. The large increase in output achieved by producing a three-way cross calf was largely a reflection of better conception rates and reduced mortality associated with breeding from a crossbred cow.

EASE OF CALVING

The only established information on ease of calving between different cow breeds is for the British Friesian. Friesian cows and crosses containing a proportion of Friesian breeding have relatively small pelvic canals in relation to their mature size and hence can be expected to have a 2 % higher incidence of calving difficulties.

MILK YIELD

Having produced a live calf, the cow must then rear it successfully, producing sufficient milk to support liveweight gains of around 1 kg per head per day with a minimum of concentrate inputs. Ideally, this requires a crossbred cow containing a proportion of either dairy or dual-purpose breeding.

EFFICIENCY OF PRODUCTION

The biological efficiency of suckled calf production can be measured as the weight of calf produced per 50 kg of cow weight maintained over the year (Table 2.3). Big cows, such as continental crosses, do produce big calves but the increase in cow size tends to require a larger input of feed than is reflected in improved calf output, hence they are biologically less efficient than medium-sized cows. However, biological efficiency is not necessarily directly associated with profitability. On farms where feed supplies are abundant and cheap, such as large arable units, the increased feed required by big cows may well cost less than the increase in calf output, making for a more profitable unit. This may well be true for both an increase in the weight of the weaned calf and also in better conformation or muscularity, an increasingly important aspect in valuing suckled calves. However, in most hill and upland units where feed is limited, it is still likely that medium-sized cows will be both more efficient and more profitable.

CONTRIBUTION TOWARDS GROWTH AND CONFORMATION OF THE CALF

As half of the growth potential and carcass characteristics of the suckled calf are derived from its mother, it is essential that the cow makes a positive contribution in this area. The

Table 2.3 Relationship between cow size and efficiency of production (MLC).

	Cow weight (kg)	Calf 200-day weight (kg)	Calf weight per 50 kg cow weight
Shorthorn cross	443	192	–
Blue Grey	450	194	22
Hereford × Friesian	472	203	–
Angus × beef breed	453	190	–
Angus × Friesian	449	193	21
Hereford × beef breed	485	194	20
Charolais × beef breed	628	239	19

increasing proportion of Holstein breeding in the national dairy herd is giving rise to concern among suckled-calf producers as to its likely detrimental effect on the conformation of calves, produced from suckler cows originating from the dairy herd. There is, however, little or no concern regarding the contribution of suckler cows originating from the dairy herd to the growth rate of their calves, the Friesian having similar growth potential to many of the exotic breeds of beef cattle (Table 2.3).

COW REPLACEMENT COSTS

Cow replacement costs can be calculated by:

$$\frac{\text{Purchase price of replacement heifers} - \text{value of cull cows}}{\text{Number of calves reared}}$$

The cost of heifer replacements is largely determined by the number available and the value of their steer counterparts. As a consequence, beef cross dairy heifer replacements are normally the cheapest.

Retaining heifers from the suckler herd as future replacements is normally more expensive. The two main factors influencing this are the increased value per kilogram liveweight of heifers bred from the suckler herd compared with beef cross heifers from the dairy herd and, secondly, the value of the steer by-product from the suckler herd. The steer calf must be commercially aceptable in its own right if the purchase price of the suckled heifer replacement does not have to include a proportion of "make-up" to allow for any price reduction associated with poor-quality steers.

The number of calves reared per cow has an obvious effect on replacement costs (Fig. 2.3). The effect of rearing an additional calf is initially large, but as more calves are reared, the difference becomes progressively smaller so that after six calves any further reduction is negligible. High cull cow values will also reduce replacement costs. In general, cull values fall dramatically, particularly once cows are over 10 years old.

The first decision in choosing a suckler cow replacement is whether it should be a beef cross heifer from the dairy herd or a suckled calf. The two types of heifer can be ranked on their ability to meet requirements of the ideal suckler cow (Table 2.4). The final choice will depend on the exact role the cows are expected to fill on any specific farm. Table 2.5 shows suitable breeds of bull for producing suckler replacements from either the dairy or suckler herd.

Although the ideal suckler cow will maximize the profitability of suckled-calf production, finding sufficient numbers at a realistic price is a major problem. Recent trends in AI figures for the UK dairy herd would suggest that the Limousin cross Friesian heifer will become the common suckler cow of

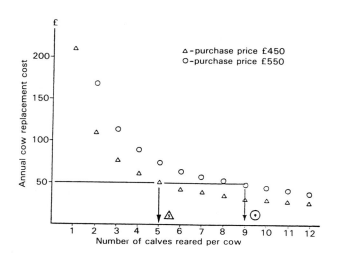

Fig. 2.3
Effect of number of calves reared per cow and purchase price on annual replacement cost/cow.

Table 2.4 Advantages of purchasing beef × dairy heifers or suckled calves as replacements.

	Beef × Dairy	Suckled
Fertility	× × × × ×	× × × ×
Ease of calving	× ×	× × × ×
Milk yield	× × × × ×	× × ×
Contribution to:		
Calf growth	× × × ×	× × × ×
Contribution to:		
Calf conformation	×	× × ×
Purchase cost	× × × ×	× ×
Cull value	× ×	× × ×
Hefting ability	×	× × × ×

Increasing × = more benefit.

Table 2.5 Breed of bull for producing suckler replacements.

	Dairy cows	Suckler cows
Aberdeen Angus	× × × ×	× ×
Shorthorn	× × × ×	× ×
Galloway	× × × ×	× ×
Luing	× × × ×	× ×
Hereford	× × × ×	×
Limousin	× × × ×	–
Simmental	–	× × × ×
Charolais	–	–

Increasing × = more benefit.

the future. Limited information from Eire on Limousin cross Friesian and Hereford cross Friesian heifers up to fifth calving in a spring-calving herd, show that there is little difference in liveweight, condition score, calving difficulty, calf birth weight, or weaning weight between the two types. The Limousin cross Friesian did however calve 7 days later than the Hereford Friesian due mainly to a delay in rebreeding first and second calvers. This suggests that Limousin Friesian crosses require slightly better feeding as heifers than do Hereford Friesians.

BREED OF TERMINAL SIRE

There is a wide choice in the breed of bull which can be used as a terminal sire in suckler herds. While the average performance of breeds of bull do differ there is more variation *within* a breed than *between* breeds. As a consequence, calving difficulties can be higher for a specific Aberdeen Angus bull, compared with another single Charolais bull! Examining the average performance of different breeds of crossing bull shows a very close relationship between the expected performance of their calves and the size or 400-day weight for the breed (Fig. 2.4).

As the size of terminal sire increases, so does the growth rate and hence sale weight of his calves. However, in addition, calf birth weight and hence the incidence of difficult calvings also increases (Table 2.6). One important aspect often ignored by suckled calf producers is that calves from larger terminal sires only grow faster by consuming more food, both indirectly in terms of increasing the milk production of their dam and directly, through consuming more supplementary feed in the form of either grass or concentrates.

Although less well documented, there is also a trend for the conformation or muscularity of calves to improve as the size of the terminal sire increases. As a consequence, suckled calves from late-maturing sires (such as Charolais, Simmental or Limousin) tend to attract a premium in terms of pence per kilogram liveweight when they are sold, reflecting the

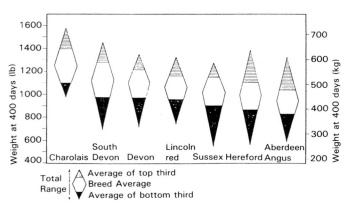

Fig. 2.4
400-Day weights for bulls from different breeds.

Table 2.6 Effects of sire breed (MLC, 1979).

	Average breed 400-day weight (kg)	Weight at 200 days (kg)			% Assisted calvings
		Lowland	Upland	Hill	
Charolais	565	240	227	205	10.1
Simmental	553	232	222	198	9.7
South Devon	544	231	221	200	8.4
Lincoln Red	500	222	214	189	6.0
Limousin	500	215	204	186	7.9
Sussex	437	215	207	186	4.0
Hereford	430	208	194	184	4.2
Angus	407	194	182	176	2.0

increasing premium being paid by the wholesale trade for carcasses of good conformation.

As a consequence of the higher growth rate, heavier sale weight and increased unit value for suckled calves sired by large breeds of bull, there has been a dramatic change in the terminal sires used in suckler herds in the past 10 years. Today the majority of terminal sires used are from the three main continental breeds – Charolais, Simmental and Limousin.

HERD MANAGEMENT

Cow nutrition is undoubtedly the most important factor influencing suckled calf production, both in terms of calf health, output and commercial viability (Fig. 2.5). Feed costs to the cow account for around 75 % of the variable costs involved in suckled-calf production for both spring- and autumn-calving herds. Current nutritional advice is based on target cow condition scores at critical points in the annual production cycle. Condition scoring is a simple, semi-objective measure of the fat reserves of suckler cows. In practice it is a good guide to the animal's nutritional status and equally important, a good predictor of her likely future performance. The critical target is the condition score at mating. In autumn-calving herds (Fig. 2.6) the target condition score is set at 2.5

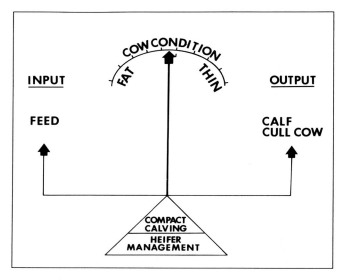

Fig. 2.5
Suckler cow
management.

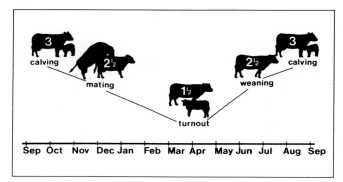

Fig. 2.6
Target condition for
autumn-calving
herds.

as cows are expected to rebreed while mobilizing body
condition on winter diets which, if sufficient to prevent
any loss of condition, become prohibitively expensive. In
comparison the target condition score at mating for spring-
calving cows is nearer 2, the high nutritive value of spring
grass allowing the cows to be in a positive energy balance
throughout the mating period (Fig. 2.7). The other aspect of
target condition scores is that they allow controlled mobilization of body reserves during the winter when feed costs are

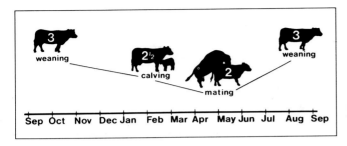

Fig. 2.7
Target conditions for spring-calving herds.

expensive. This is dependent upon body reserves being replaced during the summer from cheap energy supplies in the form of efficiently grazed grass. More detailed information on the interaction between cow condition, plane of nutrition and pattern of feeding on the fertility of suckler cows is presented by Lowman (1985).

Although attaining target condition scores for a herd allows winter feed costs to be reduced by controlled utilization of the cow's body reserves, few suckler herds are sufficiently well managed to achieve this. The problem is the wide spread of calving (the interval between the first and the last calf born in the herd) of around 5 months, which occurs in most UK herds. In this situation, with the cows being managed as one unit – the herd – feed levels have to be a compromise between the widely differing feed requirements of cows at various stages of the production cycle in the herd. As a consequence, rations are inclined to favour those cows in the herd with the highest feed requirements and, as a result, feed costs are increased.

The length of the calving period has a direct effect on conception rate. For cows calving over a 5-month period from September to January, month of calving was the largest single effect influencing conception rate and numbers of barren cows (Table 2.7). A major component of reduced fertility for late-calving cows is that they tend to be mated at their first heat post partum. On average, providing cows have not had a difficult calving, are well fed and in good condition, first oestrus will occur approximately 35 days post partum. At this point, involution of the uterus is normally complete, but in many situations the uterine environment is still non-sterile as a consequence of the previous pregnancy. Fertilization does

Table 2.7 Factors influencing fertility in autumn-calving suckler cows.

Plane of Nutrition	High	Med	Low
% conception rate to 1st and 2nd service	84	80	66
% barren cows	6	8	18
Subsequent calving interval ($\pm$ SD)(days)	358 ± 31	366 ± 33	362 ± 31
Month of calving	Sept	Oct	Nov/Dec
% conception rate to 1st and 2nd service	84	77	65
% barren cows	6	4	26
Subsequent calving interval ($\pm$ SD)(days)	378 ± 26	360 ± 30	341 ± 30

occur in the majority of cows served at their first heat post partum but when the fetus enters the non-sterile uterus a high proportion of embryonic mortality occurs, resulting in returns to service. Often the situation is further aggravated with the decomposing embryo resulting in a non-sterile uterus at second service, with the long term consequence of repeat breeders. The effect of first service at first and subsequent oestruses post calving is shown in Table 2.8. This hypothesis is supported by the analysis of 1600 records from autumn-calving herds which showed that fertility was significantly depressed if the interval between calving and the start of

Table 2.8 Effect of early post-partum breeding in autumn-calving beef cows.

First service	Number of cows	Percentage conceived
At 1st oestrus (post partum)	10	20
At 2nd oestrus (post partum)	18	78
At 3rd oestrus (post partum)	17	82

mating was less than 30 days, i.e. if the calving period was over 50 days.

A compact calving period also has a major impact on output, increasing the average age and hence the weight of calves at weaning. Herd output is further increased as a result of improved calf health and reduced mortality. Infectious diseases, noticeably scour and pneumonia, are major factors influencing mortality rates in suckled calves, after dystocia losses. In herds with a widespread calving period infectious diseases often start with late-born calves (with a low level of resistance) who are exposed to high levels of infection which are being laid down by their older, more resistant contemporaries. As a consequence, mortality rates increase as the calving period progresses (Table 2.9). In practice this trend is hidden due to the calving pattern, a high proportion of cows calving early in the calving season when calf mortality rates are low, while only a small proportion of cows calve at the end of the period when mortality rates are high. As a consequence, calf disease and mortality problems appear to be relatively constant throughout the calving period.

In order to quantify the effect of a short 2-month calving period, three commercial suckler herds were recorded as they reduce their calving period from 5 to 2 months (see Table 2.10). The overall effect of improved fertility, calf health and age at weaning resulted in an increased output of 47 kg additional weight of calf weaned for every cow in the herd — today, worth over £50 improvement in profitability for every cow.

Table 2.9 Recorded effect of month of calving on calf mortality (including calving losses) (average over three herds).

Month of birth	No. of cows calving	% calf mortality	No. of calves died
1	24	2	0.5
2	36	4	1.4
3	18	5	1.4
4	12	12	1.4
5	10	25	2.5
Overall calf mortality		7.2	

Table 2.10 Effect of sequence of calving on herd performance.

Month of calving	% Cows calving/month		Weaning %	Calf weaning weight (kg)	Weight of calf weaned/cow	
	(5 months)	(2 months)			(5 months)	(2 months)
1	24	72	98	320	–	
2	36	28	96	300	–	306
3	18	–	92	260	258	–
4	12	–	88	220	–	+47
5	10	–	75	180	–	–

One way to convince farmers of the importance of a compact calving period is to set a simple exercise (Table 2.11), with farmers supplying the cash value of cattle and feeds. The exercise is based on a 100-cow autumn-calving herd which currently has a 17-week calving period. During the winter mating period the herd is fed *ad libitum* silage supplemented with 2 kg per cow per day of concentrates. When mating is finished, concentrate supplementation stops and the cows remain on *ad libitum* silage for the remainder of the winter period. Ten cows calve during the last 7 weeks of the calving period, the balance, 90 cows, calving in the first 10 weeks. The farmer decides to reduce his calving period from 17 to 10 weeks by culling the 10 late-calving cows and replacing them with 10 early-calving heifers. This will increase the average age of all the calves in the herd at weaning by 16 days.

For the exercise, four factors are considered:

(1)   The price obtained for 10 pregnant late-calving cows of various ages (£550).
(2)   The increase in calf weaning weight due to the calves being 16 days older and the value of 1 kg of calf liveweight at weaning (16 kg at £1.20/kg = £19.20).
(3)   The value of concentrates saved due to reducing the mating period by 7 weeks (2 kg of concentrates per cow per day for 7 weeks for 100 cows = approximately 10 t concentrates) (value of 1 t of concentrates = £120).
(4)   The price the farmer can afford to pay for in-calf heifers and break even.

In Table 2.11 the farmer valued the 10 late-calving cows at £550 per head, a total income of £5500. He assumed a liveweight gain in the calves of 1 kg per head per day to give an increase in weaning weight of 16 kg per calf which, at a value of £1.20, increased calf value by £19.20/head. For 100 calves this gave an increased income of £1920. The concentrates were valued at £120/t to give an additional saving of £1200. The total income from the exercise due to selling cows and heavier calves and saving feed costs was therefore £8620. To break even, all this money could be allocated towards purchasing 10 early-calving heifers – at a price of £862 per in-calf heifer. In subsequent years the farmer would continue to save concentrates by maintaining a short mating period and also continue to have increased calf weaning weights – a total increased income of £3100/year or £31 for every cow in the herd.

In practice, with farmers supplying their own prices to determine what they can afford to pay for in-calf heifers, this simple exercise is certainly a powerful way of convincing them of the importance of a short compact 2-month calving period. The exercise assumes that having achieved a compact calving period it can then be maintained with good management. Perhaps the most crucial aspect in maintaining a compact calving period is improving the management of first calved heifers. Correct management of heifer replacements is a complex but crucial aspect of successful suckled-calf production.

Table 2.11 A simple exercise to show the importance of a compact calving period.

	Income (£)
Selling 10 late-calving cows	5500
Increased income from 100 calves	1920
Saving in concentrate costs	1200
Total	8620
Price for buying in-calf heifers to break even = £862/heifer	

CONCLUSIONS

Like any business, suckled-calf producers have to balance their costs (which are mainly the costs of feeding the cow) against output, (which is mainly the value or weight of calf produced for every cow in the herd) to ensure a profitable enterprise. This control of the enterprise can only be achieved if cows are all at a similar stage of production, i.e. that the herd has a compact calving period.

The maintenance of a compact calving period is dependent upon good heifer management – the cornerstone of a successful herd. Having achieved this, day-to-day management is based on assessing the condition of the cows in relation to the targets of the system and reacting accordingly. If feed inputs are excessive, cows will respond by becoming overfat. More commonly, if feed inputs are below requirements, cows will respond by becoming lean and failing to achieve target condition scores. If producers ignore this clear message the cow will eventually respond by failing to rebreed, resulting in financial disaster.

REFERENCES

Baber, P. L., Rowlinson, P., Willis, M. B. & Chalmers, A. J. (1984). A comparison of Canadian Holstein cross British Friesian and British Friesian steers for beef production. *Animal Production* **38**, 407–415.
Lowman, B. G. (1985). Feeding in relation to suckler cow management and fertility. *Veterinary Record* **117**, 80–85.
Wright, I. A., Rhind, S. M., Russel, A. J. F., Whyte, T. K., McBean, J. & McMillen, S. R. (1987). *Animal Production* **45**, 395–402.
Meat and Livestock Commission (1979). *Beef Yearbook*.
Meat and Livestock Commission (1981). *Beef Yearbook*.

CHAPTER 3

Vetting Compound Feeds for Dairy Cows

R. GORDON HEMINGWAY

INTRODUCTION

This chapter is concerned essentially with the evaluation of purchased compound feeds or simple mixtures of straight concentrates for dairy cows given grass silage. Readers should perhaps first consult the article by Webster (1984).

Table 3.1 details the nutrient requirements of lactating cows. The production needs, at a yield of 30 kg milk, account for 70 % of the total energy and 80 % of the total digestible crude protein needs. The first inquiring step must therefore be to confirm that the amounts of compound feed given are indeed what the farmer intends. Feeds are usually allocated on a volume basis, and scoops and buckets are frequently and notoriously wide of the mark. A recent survey of the accuracy of compound feed dispensers in milking parlours showed that half were inaccurate to the extent of 10 % either way and as many as one-quarter (of 259 farms) were out by as much as 25 %.

Where compound feeds, as opposed to straight ingredients, are used the farmer must have the confidence to trust that the manufacturer has both the expertise and the intention to provide a material which will fulfil the implied purpose. Many claims will be over-optimistic, e.g. a "4 lb/gal (0.4 kg/kg) compound" should contain 5 megajoules metabolizable energy (MJ ME). This implies 12.5 MJ ME/kg on an as-fed fresh matter basis or 14.4 MJ ME/kg of dry matter. None of the normal compound feed ingredients (except fat) contain this concentration of energy, and mineral inclusion dilutes other ingredients. The most closely guarded secret of any compounder is the ingredient formulation, and it may change continuously according to prices and availability of ingredients. It is to all intents impossible for a farmer or his veterinary surgeon to obtain even an approximation of the construction of a feed in question. Microscopic examination is a uniquely expert field and certainly not for the amateur.

The only information available to the farmer and the veterinary surgeon is the magical data on the bag for oil, crude protein, crude fibre and (more recently) ash. No account need be taken of digestibility, the type of fat, the source of fibre, the nature of the protein or the useful ingredients (or otherwise) of the ash. Added fat may reduce fibre digestibility and proteins of equal digestibility may degrade differently in the rumen. No real help is given on the appropriateness of a particular compound for use with different background diets, be they good or indifferent silage, combinations of hay and silage, or whatever. It is perhaps unrealistic to expect some indication of the way in which compound feed intake may reduce full voluntary intake of silage, but some substitution inevitably occurs and the cow is interested in the total picture.

PREDICTION OF ME CONTENT

The standard approach to the determination of the ME value of feeds is to assess the digestibilities of their components and the energy losses as urine and methane using wether sheep. Normally the sheep are fed for maintenance. This technique is open to the criticism that cows in early lactation are frequently fed at three to four times maintenance (Table 3.1). This affects rate of passage and further differences may arise in the change from milled feeds (sheep in cages) to long roughages more normally consumed by cows.

The Feed Evaluation Unit of the Rowett Research Institute conducted detailed investigations between 1975 and 1984 into

Table 3.1 Metabolizable energy (ME), digestible crude protein (DCP), rumen degradable protein (RDP) and rumen undegradable protein (UDP) requirements of a 600 kg Friesian cow.

	ME MJ	DCP g	RDP g	UDP g
Maintenance	62	350	430	nil
M + 10 kg milk	111	850	815	65
M + 20 kg milk	161	1350	1210	320
M + 30 kg milk	210	1850	1615	565

Notes:
  (1) Add or subtract 9 MJ ME for each 100 kg liveweight above or below 600 kg.
  (2) 0.5 kg liveweight loss per day in early lactation can contribute 14 MJ ME.
  (3) 0.5 kg liveweight gain per day in mid or late lactation or for growth requires an additional 17 MJ ME.
  (4) Add 3.5 MJ ME per 10 kg milk with 4.0 % fat and 8.9 % solids not fat.
  (5) Add or deduct 150 g RDP for cows losing or gaining 0.5 kg liveweight per day.

the ME values of a range of straight feeding stuffs (Table 3.2). There are considerable differences between the previously accepted values (Ministry of Agriculture, Fisheries and Food 1975, Bulletin 33, now MAFF Reference Book 433, 1984) and those obtained by the unit at the Rowett. Furthermore, all standard materials such as barley, wheat, wheat feed, soya, etc., show considerable variations from sample to sample, and the digestibility studies in wether sheep are subject to some biological error. It is not clear which values the members of the United Kingdom Agricultural Supply Trade Association (UKASTA) use in their least cost formulations and it is

Table 3.2 Metabolizable energy values of feeds (MJ ME/kg dry matter ± standard deviation) in comparison with previous MAFF Bulletin 33 (1975) values (MAFF, 1984).

	New value	Old value		New value	Old value
Barley	12.9 ± 0.9	13.7	Wheat feed	12.0 ± 1.2	11.9
Small barley	12.2	–	Wheat bran	10.8 ± 0.6	10.1
Wheat	13.5 ± 0.7	14.0	Maize gluten	12.5	13.5
Oats	12.0 ± 1.1	11.5	Peas/beans	13.5 ± 0.6	13.1
Maize	13.8 ± 0.9	14.2	Ext soya bean	13.3 ± 0.5	12.3
Manioc	12.8	12.6	Ext rape meal	12.0	10.9
Sugar beet pulp	12.5 ± 0.5	12.2	Groundnut	13.7	12.9

understood they may have their own (unpublished) data.

After 1979, the Feed Evaluation Unit, UKASTA and the National Farmers' Union arranged for the examination of 24 compound feeds of known ingredient composition (Feed Evaluation Unit, Third Report, 1981) and typical of the range of feeds for all classes of cattle. The object was to determine the ME using wether sheep and then to devise multiple regression equations based on laboratory analyses to equate with these ME values, and to assess the errors. The ingredients included *inter alia* oat feed, flour (low grade), high energy fat (blended), dry fat (50 % absorbed on a carrier), ground straw, sodium hydroxide-treated straw pellets, rice bran, cocoa bean waste, dried coffee waste, grape follicle, guar meal, feather meal and binder.

The bald statement, generally included in an undergraduate's introduction to the proximate analysis of feeds, that various combinations of old boots, string and candles will yield predetermined crude protein, fat and fibre variations, is thus not all that unrealistic. The UKASTA policy not to declare ingredients "because it would impede the introduction of new feed ingredients" seems appropriate.

EQUATIONS

From this most extensive work some 73 multiple regression equations were produced to predict ME from analytical determinations such as crude protein, crude fibre, modified acid detergent fibre, ether extract, ash, starch, gross energy, cellulose digestibility, *in vitro* digestible organic matter in the dry matter, lignin and sugar. The criterion adopted was that the residual standard deviation of the ME prediction should be less than 0.5 ME, assessed on the basis of the mean results from five laboratories. We do not all have access to five laboratories and the error is obviously greater for a single laboratory.

Other similar investigations involving digestibility trials with wether sheep have been made by Cottyn *et al.* (1984) in Belgium (32 purchased compound feeds for cattle) and Hemingway (1983) (17 "top-of-the-range" dairy feeds from 11 companies). More recently a joint UKASTA/Agricultural Development and Advisory Service working party and the

Scottish colleges have re-examined the Feed Evaluation Unit's 1981 data in the light of current formulations in the feed industry (Alderman, 1985) with a view to producing equations "suitable for EEC legislation to declare energy values".

The most successful equations leading to the lowest residual standard error were those which involved either an *in vitro* or *in vivo* assessment of digestible organic matter in the dry matter (DOMD), e.g.

$$ME = (0.142 \times in\ vitro\ DOMD) + (0.416 \times oil\ \%) - 0.11$$
(Feed Evaluation Unit, 1981)

$$ME = (0.175 \times in\ vivo\ DOMD) + (0.193 \times oil\ \%) - 1.42$$
(Hemingway, 1983)

In vitro determinations are time consuming and the numerical data obtained are very laboratory dependent. *In vivo* estimations are clearly impracticable on a large scale. Examples of equations based on proximate constituents only, and so which take no account of digestibilities of ingredients, are on a dry-matter basis:

$$ME = 13.66 + (0.261 \times oil\ \%) - (0.171 \times crude\ fibre\ \%) - (0.183 \times ash\ \%)$$
(Feed Evaluation Unit, 1981)

$$ME = 11.1 + (0.224 \times oil\ \%) - (0.007 \times crude\ protein\ \%) - (0.0713 \times crude\ fibre\ \%) - (0.182 \times ash\ \%)$$
(Hemingway, 1983)

$$ME = 11.78 + (0.065 \times crude\ protein\ \%) + (0.0665 \times oil\ \% \times oil\ \%) - (0.041 \times oil\ \% \times crude\ fibre\ \%) - (0.118 \times ash\ \%)$$
(Alderman, 1985)

It is interesting to note, e.g. Hemingway (1983), that the contribution to total ME of, say, 5 % oil is counterbalanced by the presence of either 7 % ash or 7.5 % crude fibre, all of which are common levels in present-day dairy feeds.

It should be remembered that fats contain about 2.25 times more gross energy than other ingredients of feeds, and ash has no energy. While a variation of about 0.5 MJ ME either way may be helpful in distinguishing the poorest cattle feed from the best dairy feed, it is not particularly useful in differentiating between two feeds of apparently comparable

composition. Unfortunately, the single laboratory error encountered in all these equations is of that order.

The report of the Feed Evaluation Unit indicated that its
equations should only be used within the parameters of the
constituents and proximate analyses of the 24 feeds examined.
In particular, only two had oil values above 5.0 % (fresh-matter
basis). In contrast, all the feeds examined by Hemingway (1983)
had 5.0 % oil or more (and nine of the 17 had 6.0 % oil or
more) as declared. This is important because unless fat is
protected in the rumen, the digestibility of fibre is reduced.
Also, not all fats are similar in composition. Certainly the
feeds examined by Hemingway (1983) were more typical of
current-day production (i.e. about 5–6 % oil and 7–9 % fibre)
of dairy feeds than those evaluated by the Feed Evaluation
Unit from about 1978 to 1981.

Equation U1

The best equation, proposed by Alderman (1985) and referred
to as the U1 equation, may be conveniently expressed in
fresh-matter terms so that it can be used with the values for
protein, fibre, oil and ash on the bag or invoice. It is:

$$
\begin{aligned}
\text{ME (as fed)} = {} & 10.25 + (0.654 \times \text{crude protein \%}) \\
& + (0.764 \times \text{oil \%} \times \text{oil \%}) \\
& - (0.476 \times \text{oil \%} \times \text{crude fibre \%}) \\
& - (0.118 \times \text{ash \%})
\end{aligned}
$$

Residual standard deviation = ± 0.28 MJ ME)

Equation U1

It is interesting, and embarrassing, to apply equation U1 to a
compound devised from the feeds with well-authenticated
ME values, as in Table 3.3. For example, a compound formed
from 20 % barley, 20 % wheat, 10 % manioc, 15 % maize
gluten, 15 % soya, 10 % peas, 5 % wheat feed and 5 %
minerals, would have (on a dry-matter basis) 2.0 % oil, 19.4 %
crude protein, 6.1 % crude fibre and 8.2 % ash and an ME
value of 13.0. Use of the U1 equation gives an apparent ME
of 11.8 and is clearly well wide of the mark.

The equation U1 has been applied to a range of dairy feeds
currently produced by a major national manufacturer and
compared with the oil/fibre/ash equation of the Feed Evalu-

ation Unit (Table 3.3). On a dry-matter basis equation U1 tends to give rather higher ME values at the top end and perhaps a tendency to lower values at the bottom end. It should perhaps be remembered that the Feed Evaluation Unit report stressed that its data (which are the same as that in equation U1) should not be extrapolated to high-fat feeds. The U1 equation may not be applicable for feeds with a low content of oil and a high content of digestible fibre (e.g. sugar beet pulp). Whatever the qualifications of equation U1, it lacks the necessary precision in that it cannot statistically separate feeds which are less than 0.75–1.0 MJ ME apart.

If it is accepted that these equations give ME values more or less in the current order of magnitude, the idea of a 4 or even 3.5 lb/gal cake (i.e. 0.4 or 0.35 kg/l) is, in present-day circumstances, well wide of the mark. On an "as fed" basis the range of rates of feeding to provide 5 MJ ME would be (from Table 3.3) from 0.43 kg (feed 1) to 0.51 kg (feed 5)/kg milk. Hemingway (1983) concluded that the better half of the 17 top-of-the-range dairy feeds examined should be given at rates between 0.45 and 0.50 kg/kg milk.

It appears that this conclusion may be in accord with current practice. A survey of the rate of feeding of compound feeds over the whole year by a national company based on information from over 2000 costed herds shows a steady, progressive increase from 0.28 kg in 1963 to 0.34 kg/kg milk in 1982. Other than at yields over 7000 kg per annum the

Table 3.3 Application of proposed legislative equation (U1) to predict ME values of five different milk production feeds (MJ) from one national manufacturer in comparison with Feed Evaluation Unit (FEU) equation.

Feed	Oil %	Fresh matter (as fed) basis 87 % dry matter			ME (U1)	Dry-matter basis	
		Protein %	Fibre %	Ash %		ME (U1)	ME (FEU)
1	6.0	20	7	7	11.5	13.2	12.8
2	5.5	18	7	7.5	11.0	12.6	12.5
3	5.25	16	7.5	7.5	10.7	12.2	12.4
4	5.25	18	9	8.7	10.4	12.0	11.9
5	5.0	16	9	9.9	9.9	11.4	11.6

feeding rate seemed to be independent of yield. On many farms concentrates may be given in amounts judged necessary to maintain yields, and the trend seems to be markedly upwards. With presumed advances in nutritional knowledge and the improvement in grassland and silage management over the last 20 years, the trend might have been expected to be in the reverse direction.

EVALUATION OF THE PROTEIN

In spite of its limitations (Webster, 1984) digestible crude protein (DCP) rather than rumen degradable (RDP) and undegradable protein (UDP) is still the official method of expressing protein requirements.

From digestibility trials with wether sheep using 17 top-of-the-range compounds for dairy cows, Hemingway (1983) found a close relationship:

$$DCP \% = (0.987 \times crude\ protein\ \%) - 4.5$$

This approximates to:

$$DCP \% = crude\ protein - 4.7$$

So an 18 % crude protein compound will have about 13.3 % DCP and a 16 % crude protein product will have about 11.3 % DCP. At a normal feeding rate of 0.4 kg/kg milk the amounts of DCP supplied will be 53 and 45 g (target 50 g). If, however, the feeding rate were 0.45 kg/kg milk the DCP supplied would be 60 g (18 % crude protein) and 51 g (16 % crude protein). It is thus important to establish the rate of feeding before deciding the desirable crude protein content of the feed.

It would be desirable to be able to vet the compound from the point of view of RDP and UDP. The theoretical grounds for suggesting that at higher yields a greater proportion of the protein intake should be undegradable in the rumen (but still digestible overall) (Table 3.1) is sound (Agricultural Research Council, 1980) but the system is not yet in practice. The reasons are the absence of a simple, repeatable technique for the determination of rumen degradability and for the assessment of rumen residence time for high yielding cows given a variety of systems of compound feed presentation during the day. Ring tests in numerous laboratories to determine UDP in standard feeds by an *in sacco* rumen technique have given alarmingly divergent results.

Experimental work gives results which are not highly convincing. Castle and Watson (1984) gave grass silage-fed cows (RDP 0.77) various mixtures of barley with soya bean and, or, formaldehyde-treated soya bean so as to have RDP from 0.58 to 0.47. There were no significant differences in silage dry-matter intake (about 9 kg dry matter), milk yield (about 24 kg), milk fat (about 3.7 %) or milk protein (about 3.1 %). Twigge and Van Gils (1984) reported the results of 21 experiments where grass or maize silage-fed cows were given enhanced amounts of UDP. The overall mean change in milk yield was 0.6 ± 0.7 kg, milk fat 0.05 ± 0.014 % and milk protein 0 ± 0.05 %. There were large individual variations between experiments and the authors pointed out that the response to additional UDP might depend *inter alia* on the effect on silage intake, the RDP also supplied, the type of silage, the constituents of the compound feed and its mode of manufacture.

In the present state of the art there seems to be no alternative to ensuring that cows receive first an adequate energy intake, backed up by a not ungenerous amount of crude protein. If urea is excluded (and there is no place for it in diets for high-yielding cows in early lactation) the range of normal ingredients should give a protein degradability of between 0.5 and 0.7 without any extra special selection of ingredients.

LIMITS OF VARIATION IN DECLARED ANALYSES

The 1982 Feedingstuffs Regulations allow some considerable variation in the declared analyses. This is quite reasonable as it is not possible for compounders to analyse all ingredients before use in a rapidly moving feed mill. Table 3.4 indicates the best and worst permitted situations for a commonly used compound feed together with the ME values calculated from the equation U1. The possible variation makes on-the-spot evaluation on the farm quite valueless and out-of-court for legislative purposes.

The extent to which variation from the declared analyses

R. G. Hemingway

Table 3.4 Permitted range in declared analyses and resulting predicted (U1) ME (MJ fresh-matter basis).

	Oil %	Protein %	Fibre %	Ash %	ME
Declared	5.5	18.0	7.0	7.5	11.0
Best situation	7.1	21.6	3.2	5.3	13.8
Worst situation	4.7	16.2	8.1	8.2	10.2

occurs is unknown, but two examples are disturbingly revealing. The intention for the 24 feeds made specially for evaluation in the Feed Evaluation Unit/UKASTA/National Farmers' Union exercise was such that all should contain between 2 and 4 % or between 5 and 7 % oil. In the event, seven of the 24 were outside these limits. All should have contained between 4 and 6 % or between 8 and 12 % crude fibre. Twelve of the 24 feeds were outside these limits. The authors commented that "the failure of the analytical results to fall inside the intended ranges was almost certainly due to discrepancies between the composition of the ingredients analysed and the values listed in the feed composition tables from which the formulations were derived". In an examination of 17 top-of-the-range feeds from 11 companies, Hemingway (1983) recorded that the overall mean declared fat level was 5.7 %. The determined mean was 4.85 % and 11 of the 17 were below the minimum permitted. In a similar way, the mean declared crude fibre was 6.28 % but 6.95 % was found, and seven of the 17 were above the legal limit. The mean declared protein content was 17.88 % but the mean found was only 16.88 % and three contained less than the amount permitted.

The bias around the declared analyses should not always lie on the least favourable side. There are, however, problems in that it is believed that all the fat in some feeds is not fully estimated by the official method of analysis. In any event all fats are not of equal nutritional potential. The main problem arises in those feeds which contain both less fat and more crude fibre than expected, and unfortunately this appears to be not an uncommon finding in practice.

CALCIUM AND PHOSPHORUS

For feeds given at 0.4 kg/kg milk, the minimum concentrations needed to meet the requirements for milk production are 0.62 % calcium and 0.43 % phosphorus. Hemingway (1983) recorded mean values of 1.06 ± 0.36 % calcium and 0.67 ± 0.11 % phosphorus (fresh matter basis) in a range of compound feeds for milk production. On average each 1.0 kg feed would provide 4.2 g calcium and 2.4 g phosphorus in excess of needs for milk to go towards any inadequacy in the silage. Silage should never be inadequate in calcium but a deficiency of about 10 g phosphorus per day would not be unusual. This would be met, on average, by about 4 kg of average compound feed and thus the general situation is not unsatisfactory.

THE POSSIBLE FUTURE

The onset of milk quotas has the hidden advantages of making farmers give more attention to the details of their management. Many will seek economy in conserving increased amounts of better-quality silage. Others may reduce compound feed costs wherever possible by giving straight feeds (plus minerals and vitamins) outside the parlour to provide up to, say, the first 15 kg milk. One possible advantage of this is that barley, brewers' grains and sugar beet pulp are defined standard products which do not change from year to year. Uncertainties remain if resort is made to more variable and less known materials such as maize gluten feed and manioc.

ADDENDUM

Since this paper was written in 1985 substantial changes have occurred in the ingredients used in compound feeds. In particular there is now a more extensive use of a range of fat and fibre sources such as to question the continued reliability of the U1 equation proposed by Alderman (1985). In recog-

nition of the changes in fat sources the Feedingstuffs Regulations were amended in 1982 to permit the use of an acid
extraction procedure for fats and oils which gives a higher
(and improved) definition of their concentration in compound
feeds.

A major joint exercise has been conducted by the Hannah
Research Institute and the Rowett Research Institute with the
cooperation of the feed trade, the advisory services and
farmers' organizations (Thomas *et al.*, 1988). With grass silage
as the background, feed evaluations were undertaken using
sheep in metabolism cages and (notably) with lactating dairy
cows. The range of ingredients was limited to allow systematic
concentration on changes resulting from the inclusion of (a)
3 % and 6 % fat added as either palm fatty acid oil, maize/soya
oil and three commonly used proprietary "dry" fat products,
and (b) 2 % and 4 % fibre added as straw, sodium hydroxide
and nutritionally improved straw or sugar-beet pulp/citrus
pulp. Almost 200 dietary treatments were assessed.

All the feeds were evaluated by a range of analytical
techniques including oil following acid extraction and cellu-
lase-digestible organic matter after neutral detergent extraction
(NCD). A series of equations was used to predict the ME from
these analyses. The most reliable and at the same time those
most conveniently available to a wide range of laboratories
was the relatively simple Equation E3:

$$ME \text{ (MJ)} = 0.250 \times \text{oil} \times 0.140 \times NCD$$

Equation E3

The root mean square error was 0.24 MJ ME. It was recommended that Equation E3 be used in preference to earlier
models. It is certainly backed by a substantial amount of
detailed animal work.

Finally, in vetting compound feeds for comparative purposes
it is essential to ascertain whether nutritive values are
expressed on a dry-matter or an actual-feed basis. The difference is very considerable and probably exceeds the error of
laboratory prediction.

REFERENCES

Alderman, G. (1985). In Haresign, W. & Cole, D. J. A. *Recent Advances in Animal Nutrition*. Butterworths, London.

Agricultural Research Council (1980). *Nutrient Requirements of Ruminant Livestock*. Commonwealth Agricultural Bureaux, Farnham Royal.

Castle, M. E. & Watson, J. M. (1984). *Grass and Forage Science* **39**, 93.

Cottyn, B. G., Aerts, J. V., Vanacker, J. M., Moermans, R. J. & Buysse, F. X. (1984). *Animal Feed Science and Technology* **11**, 137.

Feed Evaluation Unit, Rowett Research Institute, Department of Agriculture and Fisheries for Scotland. Report No 1, 1975; No 2, 1978; No 3, 1981; No 4, 1984.

Hemingway, R. G. (1983). *The Feed Compounder* **3**(10), 12.

Ministry of Agriculture, Fisheries and Food (1984). *Energy Allowances and Feeding Systems for Ruminants*. Reference Book 433. HMSO, London.

Thomas, P. C., Robertson, S., Chamberlain, D. G. *et al.* (1988). In Haresign, W. & Cole, D. J. A. (eds) *Recent Advances in Animal Nutrition*, 2nd edn, pp. 127–146. Butterworths, London.

Twigge, J. R. & Van Gils, L. G. M. (1984). In Haresign, W. & Cole, D. J. A. (eds) *Recent Advances in Animal Nutrition*. Butterworths, London.

Webster, J. (1984). *Veterinary Record* Supplement, *In Practice* **6**, 184.

Fertility

CHAPTER 4

Oestrus Detection in Dairy Cattle

PETER BALL

INTRODUCTION

Poor fertility performance is a serious, unrecognized cause of reduced efficiency in dairy herds. Many dairy farmers are satisfied with their herds' reproductive performance provided the cows have reasonable conception rates and do not show obvious signs of reproductive diseases. They fail to realize the deleterious effects that delays to service have on calving intervals and thus on profitability.

For most dairy herds, an average calving interval close to 365 days, with minimal spread, is ideal. It is worth repeating the often quoted figure of about £2 per cow per day loss in profit for every day by which the calving interval exceeds the ideal. Thus, one missed oestrus, assuming the cow is cycling normally, can cost the farmer approximately £40. This is true in spite of, and sometimes even because of, quotas. Many high-yielding cows, for example, will no longer be pushed to achieve maximum yields by means of high concentrate inputs. It is thus more feasible and more desirable to reduce their calving intervals towards the ideal of 365 days. Other require-ments, such as very tight seasonal calving patterns, or adjust-ments to the seasonality of calving because of price incentives, may override the desire for a 1-year calving interval. The aim is then for a specific calving date, rather than a perfect calving interval. Whichever of these aims is paramount, the majority of dairy herds falls far short of the ideal, with average UK calving intervals still over 390 days and many cows being culled simply because they fail to achieve the calving performance expected of them.

Studies in the UK and abroad based on milk progesterone profiles have shown that a high proportion of cows, if they are well fed and managed, are likely to be undergoing normal ovarian activity by the time it is appropriate to inseminate them. The main problem causing delays to insemination, therefore, is a failure in the manifestation and/or observation of oestrous behaviour at the correct time. When a herd of cows was observed continuously for 24 h a day, all the cows were seen in oestrus at least once during a 3-week period, although the cowman in his routine observations detected only just over 60 %. On the other hand, milk progesterone profiles have revealed that 5–10 % of cows are reported in oestrus other than around the time of ovulation. Other studies indicate that the figure may be as high as 20 %. If cows are inseminated as a result, the cost is wasted and reproductive problems (including the abortion of an already-pregnant cow) can ensue. Inaccurate detection of oestrus can therefore be as serious as failures in detection.

There is thus a lot of scope for increasing reproductive efficiency in dairy herds by improving oestrus detection rates so that opportunities for insemination are not missed, and by improving the accuracy of detection to minimize problems caused by recording "false heats". Efficient oestrus detection will help the farmer in two main ways:

(1)   By maximizing the potential of physiologically normal cows.
(2)   By drawing attention to those cows which have physiological problems and thus need prompt examination by the herd's veterinary surgeon.

CHARACTERISTICS OF OESTRUS

Not every stockman realizes that it is the cow being ridden that is on heat. An oestrous cow will encourage other cows to mount it and will stand firmly to be mounted. It will try to mount other cows but, unless they are themselves in oestrus, they will move away (Fig. 4.1). Exceptions to this occur when the mounted cow is trapped by obstacles such as fences and other cows, or if it is mounted from the front. It is helpful to look for signs that the cow has been mounted, such as ruffled hair on the rump and soiled flanks.

BEHAVIOURAL CHANGES

Other behavioural changes which are not unique to oestrus, but which may help to draw attention to the right cow, include aggressiveness and soliciting other cows to mount. A cow in heat and cows which are interested in it may lick each

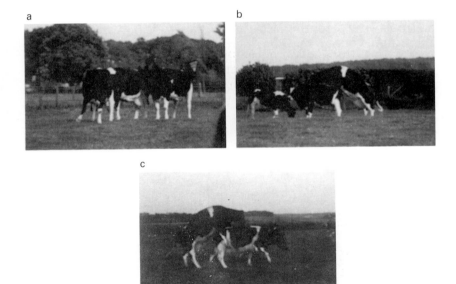

Fig. 4.1 An oestrus cow will encourage others to mount it (a) and stand firmly to be mounted (b). Unless they too are in oestrus, they will move away (c).

other, rest their chins on each others' backs and display the "Flehmann lip curl" (Fig. 4.2). The herdsman should be alert for any departure from normal behaviour in an oestrous cow and its "playmates", who may themselves be in, or close to, oestrus. The cows may, for example, be the only ones not grazing, behave restlessly and bawl, or congregate apart from the rest of the herd. They may come into the parlour later or earlier than usual, and milk let down may be inhibited in the oestrous cow.

PHYSIOLOGICAL CHANGES

Physiological changes associated with oestrus often result in the vulva becoming reddened and swollen for 1–2 days around the time of standing heat. A clear string of mucus is usually discharged from the vulva. In some cases, such as when cows are isolated or tied in cowsheds, this may be the only available criterion for insemination, but the timing relative to ovulation is more variable than that of standing oestrus. There is often a discharge of blood from the vagina 1–2 days after oestrus. Hormonal changes and/or increased activity can increase an oestrous cow's temperature and it may feel warmer to the touch and vapour may be seen rising from it on cold days.

These supplementary behavioural and physiological signs are useful in drawing attention to a cow which is in, or may be coming into, oestrus. They are not alternatives to the observation of cows standing to be mounted. This is the most reliable criterion of oestrus and the best guide to the optimum time to inseminate.

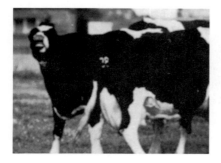

Fig. 4.2
Flehmann lip curl

IMPROVING THE EFFICIENCY OF OESTRUS DETECTION

The first step in attempting to improve oestrus detection is to make sure that the herdsman is fully aware of the importance of efficient oestrus detection. Once this priority is established, there are four main points which need emphasizing.

(1) All those who observe the cows know what to look for.
(2) Cows are observed with sufficient frequency.
(3) Adequate records are kept.
(4) Cows are clearly identified.

KNOWING WHAT TO LOOK FOR

If there appears to be an oestrus detection problem in a herd, it may be necessary to determine as tactfully as possible whether the herdsman knows exactly what to look for and whether he is giving the problem the priority it deserves. For veterinary surgeons who need to remind themselves or their clients of the basic principles, a tape/slide presentation on oestrus detection is available from the Royal Veterinary College audio visual unit.

FREQUENT OBSERVATION

Standing oestrus in a cow may persist for as little as 2 h and it is more likely to occur between 1800 and 0600 than during the day. There may well be at least 15 min between mounts. It is therefore important to watch for oestrus as frequently, and for as long, as possible. It is recommended that, in addition to milking and feeding times, when cows are less interested in oestrous behaviour, three periods of at least 20 min are set aside for observation. One of these checks should be around the middle of the day and another as late as possible in the evening. This suggestion sounds a little less unreasonable when set against the potential loss of about £40 for every missed opportunity to inseminate!

RECORD KEEPING

There are still many dairy farmers keeping virtually no records of their herd's reproductive events. It is obviously important to keep records to aid many aspects of management. It is particularly important to record oestrous events:

(1)   To draw attention to cows which have not been observed in oestrus, or which are displaying abnormal oestrus intervals.
(2)   To help decide if a suspected oestrus is genuine, by reference to previous oestrus dates.
(3)   As an aid to predicting the next oestrus date and thus increasing the chance of observing activity. Records of metoestrous bleeding, indicating that oestrus may be expected in 19–20 days, should be included.

A basic requirement is a pocket diary, which is carried at all times, so that all relevant observations can be recorded before they are forgotten. Information from the diary can be transferred to a variety of recording systems. These include rectangular wall charts and circular calendars, with or without individual cow record cards, and computer systems, either self-contained or as part of a commercial service. The recording system chosen depends to an extent on herd size and on personal preference. Various types of recording system are discussed in the MAFF reference book *Dairy Herd Fertility*.

The use of 21-day calendars to record oestrus is currently being evaluated by ADAS on smaller dairy farms (up to 55 cows) in Dyfed. Every oestrus event is recorded, the layout of the calendar being such that the date of the next expected oestrus can be seen at a glance. The calendars are useful in drawing attention to problem cows. Users should beware of being blinkered into only watching cows when the calendar shows they are due and, worse, herdsmen who have cows inseminated at the expected time, even though they are not in true standing oestrus, just to keep the record straight.

The effect of the calendars on reproductive efficiency has yet to be evaluated, but the majority of the farmers involved have found them to be a valuable aid to reproductive management.

COW IDENTIFICATION

It is often difficult to identify individual cows with certainty, especially in larger herds and where more than one man works with the cows. It is not surprising that the wrong cow is sometimes presented for insemination. Since the inseminator is not permitted to pass judgement on the fitness of the cow for insemination, the cost will be wasted and the insemination could cause problems for the cow, especially if it is already pregnant. Good, clear identification, such as that provided by an expertly applied freeze brand, is thus an important adjunct to good oestrus detection.

AIDS TO OESTRUS DETECTION

Heat mount detectors

Devices such as the Kamar heat mount detector are glued to the hair over the midline just in front of the tailhead. Pressure from a mounting cow squeezes dye from a reservoir so that a colour change is visible to the herdsman. A "triggered" detector on a cow thus indicates that it has been ridden and may be, or may have been, in heat. Specially formulated paste, applied in the same position on the cow's back, provides a cheaper alternative. In this case the paste is rubbed off by a mounting cow, thus drawing attention to a possible oestrous cow. Experimental evaluation of heat mount detectors has yielded conflicting results. Their effectiveness varies between herds, being subject to a number of factors, including the design of cubicle divisions, some of which are more likely to trigger detectors or rub off tail paste. They are likely to be useful on many farms as an aid to oestrus detection in individual problem cows.

Movement detectors

The potential of using pedometers to measure the increased activity associated with oestrus (Kiddy, 1977) was at first limited, since it was difficult to keep the devices in place on cows' legs and to read the output. Modified devices now on the market seem to offer more promise. A microprocessor in the activity monitor assesses the cow's normal level of activity. Proportional increases in activity are monitored and one of three lights on the monitor flashes according to the degree of increased activity. An attachment strap of improved design lessens the risk of the monitors ending up in slurry pits!

Closed circuit television

Relatively inexpensive systems are available for monitoring cows in calving boxes so that a herdsman can see, from the comfort of his armchair, when a cow needs attention. The cameras can also be used to monitor sexually active cows in loafing areas. Using time lapse and fast play back, a night's activities can be observed in a fairly short time. A more sophisticated system, designed especially for oestrus detection, automatically switches on for 2 min when mounting occurs. The main drawback is the difficulty of identifying cows on the screen, but trials have shown that such systems could have potential under the right conditions.

Teaser animals

In this context, teaser animals are any other animals that will mount an oestrous cow and thus draw the herdsman's attention to it. Teasers are normally other bovines, but it has been known for a billy goat to work well in this respect! Teasers can indicate that they have mounted cows by marking them with a raddle or a chin-ball marker. As a rule, the more effective a teaser animal is, the more aggressive it is likely to be, thus increasing the risk of injury to stockmen or cows. Also, if more than one cow is in heat in a herd, the teaser tends to develop favourites and completely ignore other oestrous cows. Vasectomized bulls share with entire bulls used for natural service the ability to spread venereal disease. Some preliminary work has been carried out on the possibility of using oestrogenized steers as oestrus detectors. They apparently do not penetrate when they mount, and are thus unlikely to spread venereal disease. More work is needed to assess safety aspects and their long-term effectiveness.

ALTERNATIVES TO OESTRUS DETECTION

MILK PROGESTERONE TESTS

It has been shown that reasonable conception rates can be obtained after insemination following a measured fall in milk progesterone, even when oestrus is not observed. The advent of quick, simple and inexpensive milk progesterone tests, which can be performed on the farm or in nearby veterinary laboratories, raises the possibility of using the technique in practice. Twice- or thrice-weekly sampling of an individual cow would reveal whether it was cycling, and the approximate date of ovulation. Fixed-time insemination could also be carried out in cows which are sampled daily, starting about 17 days after a previous heat, or ovulation determined by less frequent sampling. Daily sampling will determine the day on which progesterone levels fall and the cow should be served on the third day of low progesterone. It is probably advisable to use progesterone sampling in conjunction with a sound oestrus detection programme.

OESTRUS CYCLE CONTROL

Injection with prostaglandin or an analogue is a well-established means of inducing ovulation in a cycling cow. This is sometimes carried out on cows in which oestrus has been missed, and it is routine practice on some farms to synchronize groups of cows or heifers with luteolysins. This is often a good idea with groups of heifers, in which heat detection tends to be more of a problem. They are more likely to respond well to the injection than are mature cows. Even when prostaglandins are used, it is more effective to inseminate at an observed oestrus associated with the ensuing ovulation. Thus the need for oestrus detection remains and in the author's opinion it is usually better to improve the efficiency of oestrus detection than to use prostaglandin, except as a last resort in problem cows.

NATURAL SERVICE

Natural service with the farmer's own bull is accompanied by the drawbacks which artificial insemination services were set up to overcome. Two of the most serious problems are the risk of injury to stockmen or cows and the possibility of spreading venereal infections, such as *Campylobacter* species. These risks can be even greater if a bull is hired. Other likely drawbacks include restricted opportunity for genetic gain, less efficient herd management and the cost of maintaining an animal that is not producing milk. There will obviously be problems if the bull is, or becomes, infertile – especially if this is not discovered until the herd's reproductive pattern has already been disrupted.

REFERENCES

Kiddy, C. A. (1977). *Journal of Dairy Science* **60**, 235.

CHAPTER 5

Pregnancy Diagnosis in Cattle

DAVID NOAKES

INTRODUCTION

The keystone of good breeding management of cattle, and hence an important component of any scheme for monitoring or controlling herd fertility, is the accurate and early detection of pregnant and, perhaps more importantly, non-pregnant cows.

NON-RETURN TO OESTRUS

It is generally assumed that if a cow fails to return to oestrus 18–24 days after it has been served or inseminated then it is probably pregnant. Many herdsmen rely upon this as their own method of identifying pregnant cows and this is dependent upon the efficiency and accuracy of oestrus detection.

For example, consider a herd with a good average conception rate to all services of 60 %. In every 100 cows that are served or inseminated 40 should return to oestrus because they are not pregnant. However, even if the oestrus detection rate is good, at say 70 %, then 12 of the cows that fail to conceive will not be seen to return to oestrus and hence incorrectly will be assumed to be pregnant. Admittedly they may be seen to return after another oestrus cycle but this amounts to a loss of about 3 weeks.

OESTRUS BEHAVIOUR DURING PREGNANCY

About 7 % of cows show oestrus behaviour during pregnancy. While natural service is unlikely to result in the failure of the pregnancy, artificial insemination, in which the pipette penetrates the internal opening of the cervix, is likely to result in embryonic or fetal death. This emphasizes the importance of positively identifying pregnant cows so that they are not presented for artificial insemination.

THE USE OF PREGNANCY DIAGNOSTIC TECHNIQUES

In 1969 the Milk Marketing Board surveyed 767 dairy herds to inquire about their use of pregnancy diagnosis by veterinarians. Only 9.8 % of the herds had more than half their cows examined, 22.8 % had some and 67.4 % had no cows examined. The majority of animals were examined during the third month of pregnancy, although 14 % were seen after the fifth month.

A further survey by the MMB in 1979 which involved 1692 dairy farms revealed that 14.2 % had pregnancy diagnosis performed by veterinary surgeons in more than half of the cows, 43.8 % in less than half and 42.0 % had no cows examined. Of all the farms only 12.2 % had their cows examined between 6 and 8 weeks of gestation, although in those in which more than half the cows were examined, the figure was 34.9 %. In 76.8 % of all herds the examinations were performed before 4 months, the most popular time (36.8 %) being at 8–13 weeks.

In this latter survey regional variations were apparent, with the eastern region of the MMB having the greatest use of veterinary pregnancy diagnosis, i.e. 33.1 % of the herds having more than half the cows examined, and Wales the least, with only 3.4 %. Larger herds also showed evidence of greater utilization of such techniques.

METHODS OF PREGNANCY DIAGNOSIS

PLASMA AND MILK PROGESTERONE ASSAY

The presence of a normal conceptus within the uterus of the cow prevents the regression of the corpus luteum at 17–18 days after the previous oestrus and ovulation. The chances of the corpus luteum persisting in the absence of any gross pathological changes in the uterus are small, thus the presence of a corpus luteum in the ovary of a cow 18–24 days after service or artificial insemination is an indication of early pregnancy.

The corpus luteum produces progesterone which in the peripheral circulation of the cyclical, non-pregnant cow fluctuates throughout the oestrous cycle. If the corpus luteum persists because of pregnancy, then progesterone concentrations in the peripheral circulation remain elevated at the time when the cow would have returned to oestrus if it had not been pregnant (Fig. 5.1). Blood samples collected and assayed at this time can be used to differentiate between pregnant and non-pregnant cows.

Changes in peripheral blood or plasma progesterone levels are closely mirrored in milk, although the concentrations are higher with a wider margin between pregnant and non-pregnant individuals. Milk samples can be readily collected

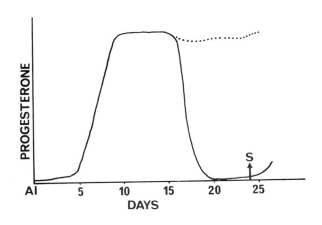

Fig. 5.1
Progesterone concentration in the peripheral circulation or milk during the oestrous cycle (continuous line) and early pregnancy (dotted line). Assuming artificial insemination at day 0, S indicates the optimum time for sampling (day 24).

by the herdsman at milking with a sample collected from each individual cow's bulked yield.

The optimum time for milk collection is 24 days after service or artificial insemination rather than 21 days. This eliminates the problem of false positive values in cows with longer than average interoestrus intervals.

The accuracy of the milk progesterone test for the positive detection of pregnant cows is about 85 %, while for the positive identification of non-pregnant individuals it is nearly 100 %. Reasons for some of the errors are as follows:

(1) Incorrect timing of artificial insemination. This is a common cause of error. If a cow is incorrectly identified as being in oestrus, but it is dioestrus (for example on day 10 of the cycle) and is inseminated, then if the cow is not observed to return to oestrus 9–11 days later and a milk sample is collected 24 days after artificial insemination it will have an elevated progesterone concentration because it will be in the next dioestrus. This is illustrated in Fig. 5.2.

(2) Prenatal death is another common reason for error although this is not a fault of the technique. The cow was pregnant at the time of sampling but there had been subsequent death of the embryo or fetus.

(3) A luteal cyst will result in persistent elevated milk progesterone concentrations.

(4) A persistent corpus luteum which gives a high progesterone level, probably associated with chronic uterine infection.

(5) A shorter than average interval between successive oestrous periods, such as 17 or 18 days, with a non-observed oestrus, will result in milk on day 24 having a progesterone concentration greater than the discriminatory level used to differentiate pregnant from non-pregnant animals.

The small number of false negative results may occur because of inadequate mixing of the milk before sampling so that a low-fat aliquot is obtained; as a result of exposure to excessive ultra-violet light; or perhaps as an error in the identification of the animal or the sample.

In the 1979 MMB survey, 4.3 % of the farms used the milk progesterone test in over half of their cows and a further 1.9 % in some of their cows. One interesting point was that

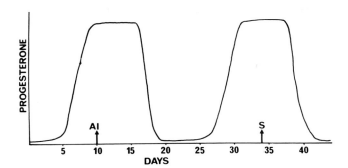

Fig. 5.2 Progesterone concentrations of the peripheral circulation or milk during two oestrous cycles. Note that if insemination is performed in dioestrus (day 10) then if oestrus is not identified around day 21 and a sample is collected 24 days after insemination (day 34, S), elevated progesterone values will be identified and the cow incorrectly assumed to be pregnant.

75 % of farms using the test also used veterinary pregnancy diagnosis.

OESTRONE SULPHATE ASSAY

Oestrone sulphate is quantitatively one of the major oestrogens in the milk of pregnant, lactating cows. During gestation the concentration increases gradually so that after day 105 it is present in the milk of all pregnant animals, whereas in non-pregnant individuals it is low or undetectable. The source of the hormone is the fetoplacental unit. The identification of oestrone sulphate in the milk of a cow of 105 days' gestation, or later, is a very reliable method of pregnancy diagnosis. However it has limited applications because of the lateness of the time that a positive diagnosis is obtained.

RECTAL PALPATION

Rectal palpation has been the standard method of pregnancy diagnosis in the cow for many years. It has the distinct advantage, compared with laboratory methods, in that an opinion can be given immediately on the farm and, if the cow is found not to be pregnant, some explanation may be given for its failure to be seen to return to oestrus and some action implemented.

Persistence of a corpus luteum

It is not possible to differentiate, on rectal palpation, between a corpus luteum of dioestrus and one of pregnancy. The presence of a full-size, mature corpus luteum about 3 weeks after a true oestrus, at which time the cow was served or inseminated, is suggestive of pregnancy.

Palpation of the amniotic vesicle

The amniotic vesicle or sac can be palpated in some cows as early as 30 days when it is about 1 cm in diameter; by 35 days it is about 1.7 cm. Those advocates of the technique, which is particularly difficult in pluriparous cows, suggest that the horn adjacent to the ovary containing the corpus luteum is gently squeezed between thumb and fingers starting at the base and extending distally to the tip. The amniotic sac is identified as a distinct, spherical, turgid object, about the size of a large pea, floating in the allantoic fluid.

Apart from the advantage of it being an early method of pregnancy diagnosis, there is little to recommend it as a routine especially because of the danger of damaging the embryo; the heart is particularly vulnerable to rupture at this stage. Subsequently, and up to about 65 days' gestation, an amniotic vesicle is more readily identifiable, feeling rather like a soft-shelled hen's egg.

Disparity in horn size and fluctuation of the uterus

The structure that is responsible for the enlargement of the uterus during early pregnancy is the allantochorion which contains the allantoic fluid. From about 30–35 days of gestation the uterine horn adjacent to the corpus luteum of pregnancy increases in size. The uterine wall feels thinner and because of the presence of allantoic fluid, it fluctuates when palpated; this characteristic is rather akin to that when a toy balloon, filled with water to the point just before the wall starts to stretch, is touched with fingers and palm of hand.

Several other factors can cause disparity in horn size, for example, poor post-partum uterine involution, pyometra and mucometra. The latter two conditions can also result in some degree of fluctuation. Twin calves distributed in each horn result in more or less equal enlargement of the horns.

Palpation of the allantochorion ("membrane slip")

From about the 35–40 days of gestation it is possible to palpate the allantochorion. This is because in a cotyledonary type of placenta the allantochorion is only attached to the endometrium at the caruncles. The uterine horn is gently grasped between thumb and either the index or middle finger and rolled and squeezed so that the contents of the horn slip away (Fig. 5.3).

The allantochorion is identified as a delicate strand of tissue which escapes from grasp just before the wall of the uterine horn. In early stages of pregnancy it is important to grasp the whole width of the horn so that the connective tissue band which runs in the allantochorion is included.

Experienced clinicians consider that it is almost an infallible method of pregnancy diagnosis, although it must be stressed that the allantochorion can persist for a short period after embryonic/fetal death (with resorption of fetal fluids) has occurred. Inexperienced persons can mistake the slipping of

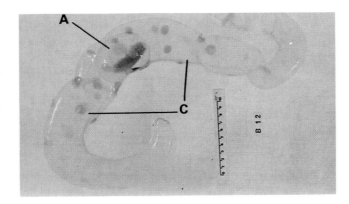

Fig. 5.3
Bovine conceptus at about 50 days of gestation. A, Amniotic sac; C, connective tissue band.

the broad ligament if it is grasped together with the uterine horn. Trying the method on fresh gravid uteri obtained from the abattoir is an excellent way of confirming what happens in this technique.

Fetal palpation

Once the amniotic sac looses its turgidity, from about 65 days of gestation, it is possible to palpate and ballot the fetus directly. Initially it feels like an amorphous floating object but eventually fetal structures can be identified.

Palpation of the caruncles/cotyledons

Except for the immediate post-partum period palpation of the caruncles/cotyledons is diagnostic of pregnancy. These can be first identified from about 70–80 days of gestation particularly in the uterine body and base of the gravid horn close to the midline, cranial and ventral to the pelvic brim; initially they canot be identified as discrete structures.

As pregnancy proceeds the caruncles grow but the size is variable depending upon the total number and their situation in the uterus.

Hypertrophy and fremitus of the middle uterine artery

It is frequently difficult to identify the middle uterine arteries in the non-pregnant and early-pregnant animal. However, as pregnancy advances the arteries increase in size, the one supplying the gravid horn in advance of the other. As well as this hypertrophy there are also changes in the pulse character from about 90–120 days of gestation, resulting in what is described as fremitus in which the artery is felt to be vibrating at high frequency.

The opposite artery usually develops the same change in pulse from about 150 days, although there is considerable variation depending upon their relative contributions to the blood supply of the uterus. In twins, where there is a fetus in each horn, fremitus develops at the same time in each artery.

The middle uterine artery, which should not be confused with the iliac, is a tortuous, mobile vessel running in the broad ligament and readily identified running ventrally and cranially close to the base of the ilium and pelvic brim. The iliac is firmly attached to the shaft of the ilium.

This method provides a particularly useful positive sign of pregnancy in large cows, such as the Charolais and Holstein, where palpation beyond the pelvic brim is difficult and retraction of the uterus impossible. Some clinicians estimate gestational age by assessing the diameter of the vessels.

Disappearance of the uterus

From about 3–5 months of gestation (longer in heifers and shorter in pluriparous cows) the uterine horns disappear out of reach over the pelvic brim and into the posterior abdomen; this is because of the weight of the fetus and fetal fluids. Although the "absence" of the uterus and the tension on the enlarged cervix are useful indications of pregnancy, positive signs such as the presence of caruncles/cotyledons and the enlarged middle uterine artery are much more reliable.

ACCURACY OF RECTAL PALPATION

Whatever method of pregnancy diagnosis is used it must have a high degree of accuracy. Surprisingly few critical studies have been undertaken to assess the accuracy of rectal palpation and in some of them the cows have been examined relatively late, i.e. at 65–70 days. However, when the method is compared with failure of cows to return to oestrus, and the milk progesterone assay, it is the most accurate, probably over 95 %.

REASONS FOR ERROR BY RECTAL PALPATION

Failure to retract the uterus and identify one positive sign of pregnancy

In large pluriparous cows the uterus is frequently situated well over the pelvic brim in the posterior abdomen and hence out of reach. Examination of the uterus for signs of pregnancy requires that it is retracted. Failure to do this and to elicit at least one positive sign of pregnancy can result in error. For this reason the diagnosis of pregnancy at 8 weeks or less is easier because retraction of the uterus is not as difficult as in later stages of gestation.

Confusion with the poorly involuted uterus

Delayed uterine involution in cows that are inseminated early after calving might give rise to the false positive diagnosis of pregnancy because of disparity in horn size. However, the uterine wall is thick and there are no positive signs of pregnancy.

Pyometra

There is always a possibility that pyometra will be confused with pregnancy (Fig. 5.4). Although the uterus is filled with fluid and fluctuates on palpation, and there is a corpus luteum present on one ovary, the uterine wall is usually thicker than that found during pregnancy when the uterus is of similar size and has a distinct "doughy" feel. Furthermore there are no positive signs of pregnancy such as palpation of the allantochorion (membrane slip), amniotic sac or caruncles.

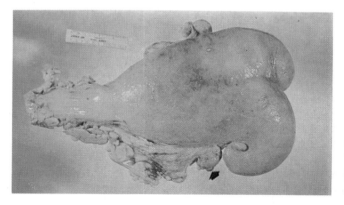

Fig. 5.4
Pyometra: note the presence of a corpus luteum in the right ovary (arrow).

Mucometra

Mucometra is a relatively uncommon condition which can be confused with pregnancy because of the presence of fluid filled uterine horns which fluctuate when palpated. In nulligravid heifers it is associated with a persistent hymen or segmental aplasia of the distal tubular genital tract thus allowing the accumulation of uterine secretions. It can also occur in cows with chronic cystic ovarian disease when the uterine wall becomes almost wafer-thin. No positive signs of pregnancy as described above under pyometra will be found.

Subsequent prenatal death

Cows may be correctly diagnosed as being pregnant by rectal palpation but the pregnancy may subsequently fail. Most embryonic deaths occur before the date of return to oestrus; however, one survey has suggested that the incidence of prenatal death between 20 and 80 days of gestation may be almost as large as that before 20 days. The later pregnancy diagnosis is performed, the smaller the error because of prenatal death. After 60 days it is probably 1 % or less.

Incorrect service date

Sometimes a cow is diagnosed as being not pregnant because of an incorrect service date, particularly when it has returned to oestrus, and has been served again perhaps 3 weeks later without this being recorded. Hence at the time of the rectal palpation the cow was pregnant, but below the minimum gestational age for a positive diagnosis to be made.

CAN RECTAL PALPATION CAUSE PRENATAL DEATH?

Concern is sometimes expressed that rectal palpation can induce embryonic or fetal death. There have been several studies to evaluate the risks, either by recording if a cow failed to calve having previously been diagnosed as being

pregnant by rectal palpation or, more recently, in association
with milk progesterone assays.

The results have been equivocal but although it is possible
that certain methods and certain individuals may increase the
incidence of prenatal death, it is likely that the rectal palpation
of cows at 41–45 days of gestation is a safe and reliable method
when performed carefully and skillfully. In those cows where
the pregnancy failed, it would probably have occurred irrespec-
tive of the procedure used. Furthermore, in experiments where
attempts have been made to induce abortion by damaging
the fetus at rectal palpation, extensive trauma has frequently
been necessary.

ULTRASONIC METHODS

Three types of ultrasound have been used for pregnancy
diagnosis. The ultrasonic fetal pulse detector uses the Doppler
phenomenon in which high-frequency sound waves, emitted
from a probe, are reflected at a higher frequency when they
strike a moving object or particles, i.e. the fetal heart or blood
flow in the umbilical arteries; these are received by the same
probe. The differences in frequencies are amplified and are
then heard as distinct sounds. External and rectal probes are
used; with the latter it is possible to identify the fetal heart
at 6–7 weeks of gestation. The technique can take much longer
than rectal palpation and a high percentage of false negatives
occur.

Ultrasonic amplitude depth analysers (A-mode) using both
rectal and external probes can be used to detect pregnancy as
early as 40 days of gestation. Although a high level of accuracy
(85–95 %) has been achieved in positively identifying pregnant
cows, a large percentage of non-pregnant cows (57–87 %) was
incorrectly diagnosed as being pregnant.

Real-time (B mode) is the most effective ultrasonic method
of detecting pregnancy in the cow. Using the transrectal
approach and a 7.5 MHz transducer, pregnancy can be detected
as early as 17–18 days by an experienced person. In the hands
of the less experienced it is possible to achieve a high level
of accuracy at around 28 days. The characteristic of the image
which is indicative of pregnancy is the presence of fluid
within the lumen of one of the uterine horns. The fluid, being

allantoic and contained within the allantochorionic membrane, is identified on the image as a non-echogenic (black) area. The horns can be located and imaged in less than 1 min. The main disadvantages of the method are currently the initial cost of the equipment and the physical difficulties of using it under farm conditions. When the equipment has become more portable, and providing confirmation of pregnancy can be made accurately before 18 days of gestation, it is likely to become a popular method.

AN IDEAL ROUTINE FOR PREGNANCY DIAGNOSIS

Obviously the earlier an accurate identification of a non-pregnant cow can be made the sooner a repeat service or insemination can be given. A milk progesterone assay may be done at the time of insemination, to ensure that the cow is close to oestrus. If it fails to return to oestrus about 3 weeks later a milk progesterone assay should be done 24 days after insemination. As part of a fertility-control programme cows that are positive to this test should be examined by rectal palpation at about 42 days with a recheck at some later stage to ensure that fetal death has not occurred. Cows that are negative at 24 days or 42 days can be treated accordingly.

THE FUTURE

Current methods of pregnancy diagnosis and the times when they are applicable are summarized in Table 5.1. However, there is a need for a method of accurate detection of pregnancy even before the expected date of return to oestrus. The cow's hormonal system recognizes that it is pregnant as early as 16–17 days after conception, with the result that the corpus luteum does not regress and the cow fails to return to oestrus. Thus even at this early stage the developing conceptus produces one or more substances which act as a signal or messenger. Attempts to identify such a messenger substance, or some other material which is produced by the cow specifically in response to the presence of the developing conceptus, such as early-pregnancy factor, will continue.

Table 5.1 Methods of pregnancy diagnosis and the times during gestation when they can be used.

Length of gestation	Method
18–24 days	Failure to return to oestrus
18–24 days	Persistence of the corpus luteum
22–26 days	Milk or plasma progesterone assay
30–65 days	Palpation of the amniotic vesicle
35–90 days	Disparity in horn size and fluctuation of uterine contents
35–90 days	Palpation of the allantochorion (membrane slip)
70 days to term	Palpation of caruncles
90 days to term	Fremitus in middle uterine artery of gravid horn
105 days to term	Oestrone sulphate in milk assay
150 days to term	Fremitus in middle uterine artery of non-gravid horn

FURTHER READING

Boyd, J. S., Omran, S.N. & Aycliffe, T. R. (1988). *Veterinary Record* **123**, 8.
Koch, E., Morton, H. & Ellendorff, F. (1983). *British Veterinary Journal* **139**, 52.
Newton, J. M., Shaw, R. C. & Booth, J. M. (1982). *Veterinary Record* **110**, 123.
Paisley, L. G., Mickelson, W. D. & Frost, O. L. (1978). *Theriogenology* **9**, 481.
Pope, G. S. & Hodgson-Jones, L. S. (1975). *Veterinary Record* **96**, 154.
Reeves, J. J., Rantanen, N. W. & Hauser, M. (1984). *Theriogenology* **21**, 485.
Tierney, T. J. (1983). *Australian Veterinary Journal* **60**, 250.

CHAPTER 6

Milk Progesterone Testing as an Aid to Cow Fertility Management

BRIDGET DREW

INTRODUCTION

The possibility of using the concentrations of progesterone in milk as an indicator of pregnancy became a reality over the past decade with the introduction of a commercial pregnancy testing service by Wickham Laboratories and the Milk Marketing Board. More recently the development of an enzymeimmunoassay technique by the Ministry of Agriculture has resulted in the production of relatively simple colour change tests suitable for use in a practice laboratory or by the farmer in the convenience of his own office.

The main advantage of the enzymeimmunoassay tests are that the results are more immediately available to the herdsmen. This enables the test to be used for purposes other than the detection of pregnancy; for the confirmation of oestrus in cows over which there is doubt or the identification of non-pregnant cows, before the expected date of the first return to service.

ENZYME IMMUNOASSAY OF PROGESTERONE IN MILK

Progesterone in milk may be measured by microtitre plate enzyme immunoassay. This technique is closely related to the enzyme-linked immunosorbent assay (ELISA) procedures used in serology. In the enzyme immunoassay (see Fig. 6.1), the plastic wells of the microtitre plate have an antiprogesterone antibody attached (1). The milk samples are added to the wells, followed by progesterone labelled by linking with an enzyme. Both progesterone in the milk and the labelled progesterone can attach to the antibody on the plastic and there is "competition" for the limited number of binding sites (2). The more progesterone present in the sample the less labelled progesterone will bind and vice versa. After a suitable

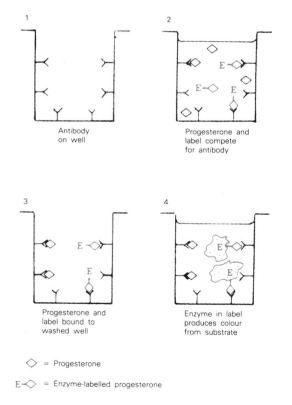

1
Antibody
on well

2
Progesterone and
label compete
for antibody

3
Progesterone and
label bound to
washed well

4
Enzyme in label
produces colour
from substrate

◇ = Progesterone

E◇ = Enzyme-labelled progesterone

Fig. 6.1
Outline steps
involved in enzyme
immunoassay of
progesterone in milk.
See text for details.

period, the wells are emptied and rinsed, leaving only such labelled progesterone as has been able to attach to the surface of the well (3). A colourless substrate is added and the enzyme in the label converts this to a coloured product (4).

In a sample from an oestrous cow, containing low levels of progesterone, more label will have been bound and a strong colour will be produced. Samples with a high concentration of progesterone arising from luteal activity will have little colour, allowing the reproductive status of the animal to be determined.

PRODUCTS AVAILABLE

There are a number of kits currently available. They vary in cost per well, the number of standards supplied, their simplicity of use and the time required to complete the assay. The most convenient and cost-effective kit to use will vary from practice to practice or farm to farm depending on factors such as the purpose of the assay and the number of samples to be assayed at any one time.

SAMPLE COLLECTION

Milk samples should be taken from the collecting jar after milking (whole mixed milk) or, if this is not possible, from one-quarter after the foremilk has been extracted. Strippings should not be used. The milk should be stored in a fridge in a carefully labelled sample bottle containing a preservative. A waterproof pen should be used to mark the number of the cow, the date and reason for sampling on the other side of the bottle.

USING THE KITS AS AN AID TO FERTILITY MANAGEMENT

The economic benefit to be obtained will depend on the level of fertility on the farm and the cost of each test undertaken.

The greatest benefit will obviously be obtained on farms where submission rates (oestrus detection) are poor or where pregnancy rates are low.

TO IDENTIFY PROBLEM COWS BEFORE SERVICE

Progesterone testing is particularly useful in seasonally calving herds where poor oestrus detection or a high proportion of non-cyclical cows is suspected.

All cows calved 21 days or more are sampled once weekly for 3 weeks (four samples) before the start of the breeding season. The results will identify problem cows and indicate which week normal cows are likely to show oestrus. An example is given in Table 6.1.

TO CHECK THAT A COW IS IN OESTRUS WHEN SERVED (Fig 6.2A)

A sample of milk taken on the day of insemination will confirm that the cow has a low level of progesterone. This procedure allows the accuracy of oestrus detection to be checked and prevents valuable semen being used unnecessarily. It will also reduce the risk of abortion in cows already pregnant and the date of the next calving can be predicted more accurately.

Table 6.1 Interpreting results from progesterone test kit.

Date sampled				Interpretation
Nov 1	Nov 7	Nov 14	Nov 21	
No colour	Colour	No colour	No colour	Normal – cow due about Nov 28
Colour	Colour	Colour	Colour	Cow not cycling?
No colour	No colour	No colour	No colour	Cow abnormal (or pregnant)?
Colour	No colour	Colour		No colour	Cow may be abnormal?

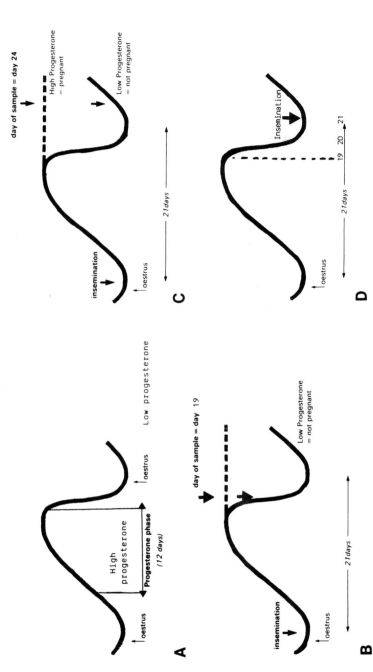

Fig. 6.2 Application of test kits in determining levels of progesterone during oestrous cycle: A, Checking a cow is in oestrus when served; B, return to service test; C, pregnancy diagnosis at 24 days after service; D, serving without oestrus detection.

DAY 19 TEST (RETURN TO SERVICE TEST) (Fig. 6.2B)

A sample taken 19 days after insemination will identify a high proportion of non-pregnant cows before return to service. The detection rate at the first return should therefore be improved. In a farm trial conducted by the Agricultural Development and Advisory Service the day 19 sample gave an accurate prediction of impending return to oestrus in 78 % of 241 non-pregnant cows sampled.

PREGNANCY DIAGNOSIS AT 24 DAYS AFTER SERVICE (Fig. 6.2C)

A colourless result from a 24 day test indicates pregnancy. A coloured result shows that the cow is not pregnant and has returned to service. Checking that the cow is in oestrus on the day of service improves the accuracy of the 19 or 24 day samples as insemination at the wrong time gives a high level of progesterone on day 24. Some cows which are pregnant when the milk sample is taken suffer early embryonic death. It is also well known that certain disease conditions lead to a "false diagnosis". For instance, metritis may cause a high level of progesterone for several weeks and cystic ovaries may also produce progesterone. Cows with either of these conditions can give a positive milk test 3 weeks after service, even though they are not pregnant.

TO SERVE WITHOUT OESTRUS DETECTION (Fig. 6.2D)

Daily samples from day 17 after last established oestrus will show the drop in progesterone as it occurs. This will indicate when the cow is in heat even if there are no visible signs. The cow should be served on the third consecutive day if the result is strongly coloured (Table 6.2).

Table 6.2 Colour changes using progesterone test kit from day 17.

Sample day	17	18	19	20	21
Result	Colourless	Colourless	Some colour	Colour	Colour

CONFIRMATION OF THE PRESENCE OF A CORPUS LUTEUM

The sampling of cows before a veterinary visit can establish the presence of a corpus luteum before injection of prostaglandin. The routine sampling and treatment of cows not observed in oestrus is proving to be a successful method of improving calving to first service intervals in a large herd with a poor record of oestrus detection. The test could also be used as an aid to diagnosis of individual cow fertility problems.

THE FUTURE

It is likely that in the near future other tests will be available which are sufficiently simple and quick to be undertaken during milking with the result available before the cow leaves the parlour. This is obviously an attractive prospect for the farmer and will mean, almost inevitably, that before long progesterone testing on farms will be in widespread use.

The veterinary surgeon in regular contact with the farm is uniquely placed to advise on the most cost-effective management for his or her client. Whether or not practices offer a testing service, encourage on-farm use or suggest a combination of both will depend on individual circumstances and preferences. Whichever method is adopted the technique provides a basis of better understanding of the problems which limit cow fertility and an opportunity for improved herd performance and liaison between the veterinary surgeon and the farmer client.

CHAPTER 7

The Individual Infertile Cow

DAVID NOAKES

INTRODUCTION

With the development of herd fertility control programmes and the tendency to measure the fertility of the herd or sub-group within a herd, sometimes the individual cow is ignored. It is axiomatic that the fertility of the herd is just a reflection of the fertility of the individual animals within the herd. Furthermore, problems identified in a few individuals may represent the "tip of the iceberg" or they may provide a warning of problems to come for the herd as a whole.

DEFINING THE PROBLEM

There is little difficulty in defining a fertile cow; it is one which gives birth to a live calf approximately every 12 months. A sterile cow is permanently unable to become pregnant and to give birth to a live calf. An infertile cow implies reduced fertility, i.e. the cow is ultimately capable of becoming pregnant and giving birth to a live calf, but the interval between successive births will be greater than 12 months; some people use the term subfertility in this situation.

Two questions arise from these definitions: First, is it possible to know if a cow is infertile or sterile? The answer is that, apart from some obvious conditions readily detectable on clinical examination, it can only be determined given time. Secondly, how long should a cow be kept so that it will eventually give birth to a live calf? The answer will depend upon the intrinsic value of the cow and the calving pattern within the herd. In the case of a valuable pedigree animal the main concern is probably the ultimate production of progeny from the cow, whereas in a commercial, seasonally calving herd there would be no merit in retaining such cows in the herd after the end of their lactation.

Whatever the decision, the fact that every day's extension of the calving to conception interval beyond 85 days is costing the farmer up to perhaps £3 per day must be taken into the equation. Furthermore, by persevering with infertile cows there is a possibility of inadvertently selecting for poor fertility in future generations.

IDENTIFYING THE INFERTILE COW

The early identification of the infertile cow is paramount. Clinical examination may identify the problem and early treatment can be implemented so that the cow can be retained within the herd and give birth to a calf after about a 12-month interval.

It is the responsibility of the herdsman to identify the infertile cow in the first instance. This will require accurate records of reproductive events (Table 7.1). He should identify the infertile cow because it is unlikely to fit the agreed herd target – in particular it is unlikely to give birth to a calf approximately 12 months after the previous one. Alternatively it may be showing abnormal reproductive behaviour – the two are not mutually exclusive.

The following cows should be examined:

(1) Those in which oestrus has not been observed after a reasonable time interval after calving.
(2) Those with repeated regular returns to oestrus after service or artificial insemination.

Table 7.1 Expectations of fertility*.

Service number	Number of cows served	Number of cows pregnant	Number of cows not pregnant	Mean calving to conception interval, days
1	100	55	45	55
2	45	24	21	76
3	21	12	9	97
4	9	5	4	118
5	4	2	2	139
6	2	1	1	160

*Assuming a 55 % chance of pregnancy at each and every service, and a mean calving to first service interval of 55 days and interservice interval of 21 days.

(3)   Those with irregular intervals to returns to oestrus after service or artificial insemination.
(4)   Those with short irregular interservice or interoestrus intervals and/or prolonged periods of oestrus.
(5)   Those with an abnormal vulval discharge.

EXAMINATION OF THE INFERTILE COW

It is important that an accurate history is obtained and a good clinical examination, particularly of the genital system, is performed (Figs 7.1 and 7.2).

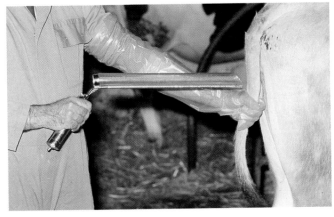

Fig. 7.1
Vaginal speculum before insertion.

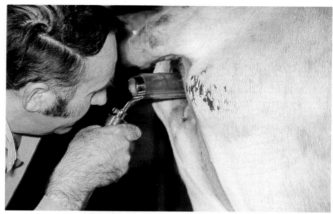

Fig. 7.2
Visual inspection of
the cervix and vagina
using the vaginal
speculum.

PROCEDURE

History

Determine the last calving date and all previous calving dates, details of the calving, and post-calving period; determine parity, current yield, feed composition and intake; the oestrus-detection regime; whether other cows are showing similar problems; natural service or artificial insemination dates and if there is a bull on the premises.

Clinical examination

Determine if the cow is pregnant or not. If there is a suspicion that it might be pregnant but it is too early to detect – leave and re-examine at a later date. Cows can conceive as early as 14 days post partum.

If the cow is definitely not pregnant proceed as follows:

(1) Check general health and determine bodily condition either arbitrarily or using a conventional body-scoring procedure.

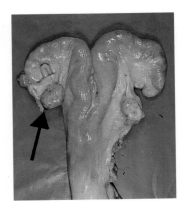

Fig. 7.3
Normal genital tract from cow in early dioestrus with a
corpus luteum on left ovary.

(2)   Examine vulva, tail and flanks for evidence of discharge.
If there is an abnormal discharge, perform a manual or specular
examination of vagina and cervix.
(3)   Rectal palpation of cervix and uterine horns to determine
if uterine involution is complete – this should be so by 42
days post partum at the very latest. Assess the degree of
uterine tone, and whether the uterine wall feels doughy and
oedematous; compare the relative sizes of the uterine horns.
Check on the absence of adhesions involving uterine horns
and broad ligaments (Fig. 7.4).
(4)   Palpate both uterine tubes for evidence of thickening or
enlargement (these are frequently difficult to identify if they
are normal).
(5)   Palpate ovaries, assess their mobility and absence of
adhesions. Determine size, shape and structures palpable. Is
there a corpus luteum palpable? Are there follicles palpable?
Is there evidence of a cystic fluctuating structure of more than
2.5 cm in diameter? Are the ovaries small, flattened, smooth
and featureless? See Figs 7.3–7.11.

Milk progesterone assay

Collect a milk sample for a progesterone assay to confirm the
nature of ovarian structures identified on palpation.

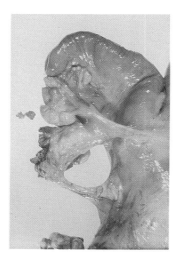

Fig. 7.4
Genital tract from cow with adhesions involving base of left
horn, uterine body, broad ligament, ovary and ovarian
bursa.

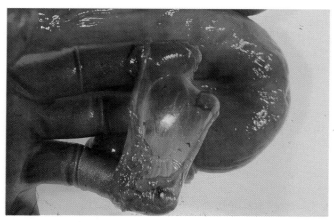

Fig. 7.5
Normal ovarian bursa
and uterine tube
(oviduct).

Other tests

Other specific tests, such as the phenol-sulphonphthalein dye
test may be considered.

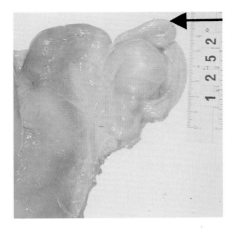

Fig. 7.6
Enlargement of the right uterine tube (oviduct) due to hydrosalphinx.

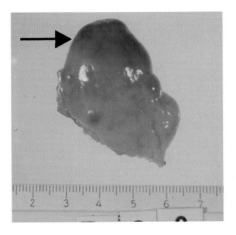

Fig. 7.7
Left ovary of cow at mid-dioestrus (day 10) with mature corpus luteum.

CATEGORIES OF INFERTILE COWS

OESTRUS NOT OBSERVED

Once a heifer has reached puberty, provided that it remains in normal health and is adequately fed, it should have repeated, regular oestrous cycles into and throughout adulthood. Only pregnancy and the immediate post-partum period should interrupt this pattern.

Most dairy cows will have their first ovulation 3–4 weeks

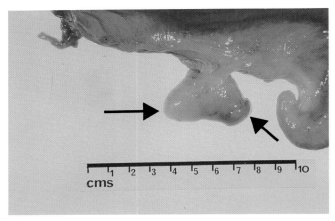

Fig. 7.8
Right ovary of cow at mid-dioestrus with mature corpus luteum and 1.5 cm mid-cycle follicle.

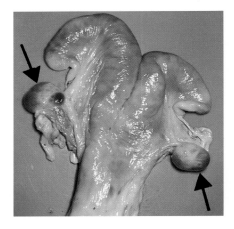

Fig. 7.9
Genital tract of cow with several follicular cysts on both ovaries.

after calving, it takes a little longer in beef suckler cows. The first post-partum ovulation frequently occurs in the absence of behavioural signs of oestrus, however, the second and subsequent ovulations nearly always occur in association with behavioural signs. A prolonged interval to the first service after calving may result in an extended calving to conception interval. Most cows should have been observed in oestrus by 42 days after calving, and, even though it is too early for service or artificial insemination, it is important that these are recorded.

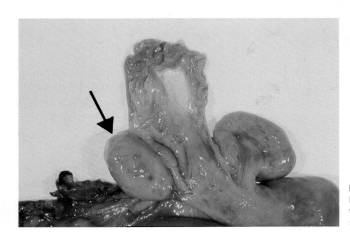

Fig. 7.10
Left ovary of cow
with no palpable
structures present.

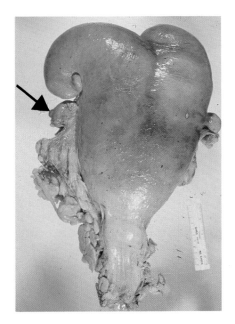

Fig. 7.11
Pyometra with corpus luteum in left ovary.

Type 1

History

Calved at least 6 weeks ago; approximately 12-month calving
intervals previously; normal calving and periparturient period;
average yield, adequate feeding; apparently a good oestrus-
detection regime; very few other cows in the herd with similar
problem; no possibility of pregnancy.

Clinical examination

Good health and reasonable bodily condition; not pregnant;
normal tubular genital tract; no vulval discharge, normal
ovaries with corpus luteum palpable. Milk progesterone concentration high.

Diagnosis

The diagnosis is given as suboestrus/silent heat, or oestrus
occurred but was not detected, or a persistent corpus luteum.

Suboestrus or silent heat has been considered to be a cause
of infertility for many years. In normal cows, apart from the
first post-partum oestrus, ovulations rarely occur in the absence
of behavioural oestrus. However, the duration of behavioural
oestrus is variable with as many as 20 % of cows being in
oestrus for less than 6 h and with some cows being mounted
just once during this period. Furthermore, behavioural signs
of oestrus are more obvious if several cows are in oestrus at
about the same time, so that when a cow is the only one in
oestrus at a particular time it may have limited opportunities
to demonstrate the fact.

If a large number of cows in the herd are involved,
particularly if there are a large number of interoestrus intervals
of 36–48 days and cows are frequently submitted for pregnancy
diagnosis when they are not pregnant, then the problem is
one of poor oestrus detection. Inquiries concerning the oestrus-
detection routine and whether the persons involved are aware
of the true signs of oestrus may confirm this diagnosis.

A persistent corpus luteum, in the absence of pregnancy, is only likely to occur if there is a uterine infection such as pyometra.

Treatment

This will depend on the time interval from calving and thus the urgency to serve the individual. Treatment with prostaglandin $F_{2\alpha}$ or analogue should induce oestrus in 2–5 days. Thus the herdsman should be warned to be extra vigilant in his oestrus detection. The simultaneous use of tail paint or a heat mount detector is frequently worthwhile. Insemination should be done at the normal time in relation to the onset of oestrus.

If oestrus is not observed, the cow should be re-examined 11 days later and a second injection of $PGF_{2\alpha}$ given followed by fixed-time insemination. A progesterone-releasing intravaginal device (PRID), inserted for 12 days with $PGF_{2\alpha}$ injected 24 h before withdrawal, is effective but more expensive.

If there is evidence that this is a herd problem due to poor oestrus detection then the following needs to be investigated and corrected:

(1) Ensure that the herdsman is aware of the true signs of oestrus.
(2) Determine the timing and routine for oestrus detection and increase the duration of observation and the frequency, if necessary.
(3) Ensure that there is adequate space and the correct environment for cows to exhibit oestrus behaviour.
(4) Use oestrus-detection aids.
(5) Routine use of milk progesterone assays.
(6) Consider using natural service.

If a persistent corpus luteum is suspected in association with uterine infection, especially pyometra, $PGF_{2\alpha}$ should be used and the cow re-examined about 7 days later.

Type 2

History

Similar to that described for Type 1.

Clinical examination

Good health and reasonable bodily condition; not pregnant; normal tubular genital tract with moderate to good uterine tone; normal ovaries rounded contour with evidence of follicular growth, no corpus luteum palpable; milk progesterone low.

Diagnosis

The diagnosis is given as suboestrus/silent heat, or oestrus not detected, or approaching first post-partum oestrus/ovulation.

The cow may be approaching the first post-partum oestrus and ovulation or a subsequent oestrus, or it may be in oestrus or going out of oestrus. Evidence of vulval mucus, especially if discoloured with fresh blood (metoestrus bleeding) will help to confirm this.

Treatment

This will depend upon the time interval from calving and thus the urgency to serve the individual. $PGF_{2\alpha}$ will be ineffective. A re-examination in 10 days (or milk progesterone assay) should be able to establish the presence of a corpus luteum and hence the presence of normal cyclical activity. If there has been a long delay since calving the use of a PRID for 8 days with $PGF_{2\alpha}$ injected 24 h before removal is probably the best treatment.

Type 3

History

Similar to that described for Type 1, except that it might be a first calver or yielding above average for the herd. It might have had some periparturient problems such as metritis, mastitis or metabolic disturbances.

Clinical examination

Perhaps poorer bodily condition than its contemporaries; not pregnant; normal tubular genital tract; no vulval discharge; ovaries small, smooth, flat with no detectable structures palpable. Milk progesterone concentration is low.

Diagnosis

Acyclic (true anoestrus) is diagnosed. Sometimes it is difficult to differentiate from the Type 2 described above. Confirmation will require a re-examination, or alternatively another low milk-progesterone concentration after 10 days. Prolonged acyclicity is uncommon in dairy cows unless they are very high yielders or fed an inadequate diet. A few animals may become acyclic having already ovulated once or perhaps twice.

Treatment

Increase food intake (if possible) and improve the quality of feed stuffs. Insert a PRID for 12 days perhaps with 600 iu pregnant mare serum-gonadotrophin injected on the day of withdrawal. Oestrus should occur within 3–4 days.

Type 4

History

Similar to that described for Type 1.

Clinical examination

Similar to that described for Type 1 except that one or perhaps both ovaries will be large (4–5 cm in diameter) and contain a fluctuating fluid-filled structure(s) greater than 2.5 cm in diameter. Milk progesterone concentrations probably high.

Diagnosis

This diagnosis is ovarian cyst(s) of the luteal (luteinized) type if milk progesterone concentration is high.

If it is a true luteal cyst it will usually have a thick wall and, because it produces progesterone, suppresses cyclical activity because of its negative feedback effect on the hypothalamus/anterior pituitary gland. Some cysts are associated with acyclicity but do not appear to secrete progesterone because milk concentrations are low. A cyst occurs as a result of anovulation of a follicle which does not regress and become atretic.

Treatment

If there is a luteal cyst, treatment with $PGF_{2\alpha}$ will cause regression with oestrus in two to three days, when the cow should be served. Non-luteal cysts can be treated with human chorionic gonadotrophin (hCG) or gonadotrophin releasing hormone (GnRH) to cause luteinization which can be followed 10 days later with $PGF_{2\alpha}$. The insertion of a PRID for 12 days will result in regression of the cyst.

Type 5

History

Similar to that described for Type 1 except that dystocia, placental retention or a puerperal metritis may have occurred. Perhaps a purulent vulval discharge, probably intermittent.

Clinical examination

Good health and reasonable bodily condition; not pregnant although the horns may be enlarged with an oedematous uterine wall; ovaries normal with palpable corpus luteum; or round with follicles as in Type 2. Purulent material in vagina seen to escape from the cervix when viewed with a speculum.

Diagnosis

The diagnosis is pyometra with retained corpus luteum (Fig. 7.11) or persistent endometritis with oestrus not observed. An enlarged, pus-filled uterus must be differentiated from a pregnant uterus, absence of "membrane slip" should confirm this but if there is any doubt, re-examination after 10 days is important.

Treatment

If a corpus luteum is present, $PGF_{2\alpha}$ will cause regression of the corpus luteum and a return to oestrus. If no corpus luteum is present the condition is probably resolving itself spontaneously, however, 3 mg of oestradiol benzoate intramuscularly might be tried.

REPEATED REGULAR RETURNS TO OESTRUS

This implies that the cow is repeatedly returning to oestrus after each service or insemination at what are considered to be normal intervals of 18–24 days. These are sometimes referred to as "repeat breeders" or "cyclic non-breeders."

When a cow is served or inseminated there is only a 60–65 % probability at the most, that it will subsequently calve to that service. This will be the same for each and every service. Nationally it is probably even less. Therefore you will see from Table 7.2 that, if a total of 100 cows are served, and assuming a 60 % probability of calving to ech service, then 16 cows will need three or more services and two cows will require at least five services to ensure that they will calve.

What are the reasons for 40 % that fail to calve to each service? In about 10–15 % of the total the oocyte is not fertilized; in about 15–20 % of the total the embryo dies at, or before, day 13 of the oestrous cycle, i.e. before the maternal recognition of pregnancy has occurred. In these individuals there will be a return to oestrus after a normal interval of 18–24 days. In about 10 % of the cases late embryonic death occurs between 14 and 42 days and in about 5 % of the total there is fetal death.

If a cow regularly returns to oestrus after a normal interval, then it means that either fertilization is not occurring or early death of the embryo (before day 13) is occurring.

History

Cow calved about 4 months ago; regular return to oestrus after the last three services; normal calving and normal periparturient period (or severe dystocia with placental retention and post-partum metritis); approximately 12-month calving intervals previously; average yield, adequate feeding; very few other cows with similar history.

Clinical examination

Good health and reasonable bodily condition; not pregnant, normal tubular genital tract (or extensive adhesions involving both horns, broad ligament and uterine tubes); normal ovaries showing evidence of normal cyclical activity (or ovarobursal adhesions); no abnormal vulval discharge.

Table 7.2 Reasons for cow failing to calve after each and every service.

Assuming that ovulation occurs and that there is a 50–60 % calving rate to each service. The reasons for the 40–50 % of services that fail to result in a cow calving at term are that:

In 10–15 % of total the ovulated oocyte is not fertilized
In 15–20 % of total early embryonic death occurs before the time of maternal recognition of pregnancy (about day 13)
In 10 % of total late embryonic death occurs after the time of maternal recognition of pregnancy (about 13–42 days)
In 5 % of total fetal death occurs (after day 42)

Diagnosis

In most cows a precise diagnosis cannot be made in the absence of detectable lesions. A normal cow may well become pregnant at the next service or there may be repeated fertilization failure (especially if there are severe pathological lesions palpable on rectal examination), or there may be early embryonic death. Other tests can be used to improve the diagnosis but these are rarely justifiable economically: patency of the uterine tubes can be assessed using the phenol-sulphonphthalein dye test. While it would be possible to determine if fertilization was occurring by attempting to recover an embryo or degenerating unfertilized oocyte at 7–8 days after service.

Fertilization failure

The failure to achieve fertilization can be due to several factors.

Acquired lesions involving the ovary, ovarian bursa, uterine tubes and uterine horns which either completely occlude the tubular genital tract, or interfere with the transport of gametes resulting in fertilization failure. There is no treatment.

Anovulation where the mature follicle fails to ovulate and regresses. Waves of follicular growth with regression occur throughout the oestrous cycle, however, normally after oestrus one follicle will ripen and ovulate liberating the oocyte. This is most likely to occur during the early post-partum period when, occasionally, luteinization of follicles occurs. These structures behave rather like a corpus luteum with regression and return to oestrus.

Diagnosis only can be determined by sequential rectal palpation, as no corpus luteum will be formed, or by milk progesterone assays; although luteinized follicles could not be distinguished from corpus luteum because both would produce high progesterone concentrations.

If this is believed to occur repeatedly GnRH or hCG can be used at the time of insemination.

Delayed ovulation, where the follicle ovulates later than the normal time of 12–15 h after the end of oestrus. Spermatozoa start to show reduced capacity to fertilize by about 15–20 h after insemination thus, if ovulation is delayed, they may well be incapable of fertilization.

Diagnosis can be difficult unless sequential rectal palpations are performed to detect the time of ovulation.

If this is believed to occur repeatedly then GnRH or hCG can be used at the time of insemination, or a second insemination can be given 24 h after the first one.

A hostile uterine environment can be spermicidal, it can also interfere with sperm and egg transport. The most likely cause would be an endocrine imbalance caused by asynchrony of some of the hormonal changes that occur during the oestrous cycle.

Rational treatment is not practicable because it is impossible to determine the precise cause. Chronic uterine infection would provide a hostile environment, although it is unlikely that infection would persist in a cow that has been calved 4 months and has undergone normal cyclical activity, unless there was a specific problem such as a pneumovagina.

Early embryonic death

Early embryonic death can be a result of a variety of factors.

Nutritional deficiencies or excess, which probably exert their effect by producing a hostile uterine environment. This is most likely to be a herd problem rather than in a single or small number of cows, except for first calvers and high yielders.

Endocrine deficiency and imbalance is probably an important cause but it is difficult to prove. Luteal deficiency resulting in reduced progesterone production by the corpus luteum has been suggested as a cause. Human chorionic gonadotrophin which is luteotrophic, and progesterone supplementation have been used.

Infection can create a hostile environment for the early embryo, however, it is most unlikely that non-specific infection would persist so long after calving because of recurrent oestrous cycles.

Genetic incompatibility is difficult to prove. Changing the sire if it has been used repeatedly is worthwhile or perhaps use a different breed.

Stress is a possible cause, but it is difficult to prove.

Fatty liver disease occurs in cows that are over-fat at calving and are subsequently fed insufficient energy for their productive requirements thereafter. This condition can be prevented by good attention to feeding practices during late gestation and after calving.

AN EMPIRICAL APPROACH TO THE REPEAT-BREEDER COW

In most cases a specific explanation for the repeated return to oestrus after service cannot be determined. Frequently, if cows are given adequate time, they may ultimately conceive. An empirical approach can be used, one such approach is as follows: The cow is inseminated at the normal time, when hCG (3000 iu, intravenously) or GnRH is used, a repeat insemination is given 24 h after the first, in both cases a bull of a different breed is used. Alternatively, natural service can be used followed by artificial insemination the next day. Human chorionic gonadotrophin (4500 iu, intramuscularly) is then given on day 13 of the oestrous cycle to boost luteal function.

IRREGULAR INTERVALS TO RETURNS TO SERVICE

The intervals are greater than 24 days and may reflect management faults associated with failure to detect oestrus, or the incorrect identification of oestrus, or late embryonic, or early fetal death.

History

Normal calving, about 4 months ago; approximately 12-month calving intervals previously; adequate feeding; returned to oestrus two to three times with intervals exceeding the normal of 18–24 days.

Clinical examination

Good health and reasonable bodily condition, not pregnant; normal tubular genital tract and normal ovaries showing evidence of normal cyclical activity; perhaps in some animals a possibility of an abnormal vulval discharge.

Diagnosis

The diagnosis is given as one or more oestruses not detected, or incorrect detection of oestrus or late embryonic/early fetal death. One missed oestrus will result in an interval of 36–48 days, two missed oestruses will result in an interval of 54–72 days. Treatment is the same described for cows with non-detected oestrus Types 1 and Types 2.

An incorrect detection of oestrus, when the cow is in fact in dioestrus, may be a result of mis-identification of the cow or reliance on the mounting behaviour as a sign of oestrus. If it is a single mistake then examination of the adjacent intervals will show that one of them will be less than normal and the sum of the long and short interval will be a multiple of 18–24, e.g. the long interval might be 32 days and the previous interval might be 10 days. If there are repeated mistakes then there will be repeated irregular intervals. Treatment is the same as described for non-detected oestrus Types 1 and 2.

Late embryonic or early fetal death will be due to the same reasons described for the cow with repeated regular returns to oestrus with early embryonic death. If numbers of cows have a similar history and if there is evidence of a vulval discharge, diseases such as *Campylobacter fetus* infection or genital infectious bovine rhinotracheitis should be suspected.

SHORT IRREGULAR RETURNS TO OESTRUS AND/OR PROLONGED OESTRUS

Normally, behavioural oestrus lasts on average 15 h with a few cows extending for as long as 30 h.

History

Calved at least 4–5 weeks ago; normal calving and periparturient period; average yield, perhaps fallen recently; adequate feeding; apparently in oestrus for several days every 7–8 days, although the main behavioural sign is that of persistent and indiscriminate mounting of other cows (nymphomania). The oestrus-detection regime for the rest of the herd has been somewhat disrupted.

Clinical examination

Good health and reasonable bodily condition; not pregnant; clear water mucoid vulval discharge; uterine horns show moderate tone; one or both ovaries enlarged at least 5 cm in diameter with several thin-walled fluid-filled structures greater than 2.5 cm in diameter. Milk progesterone concentration is low.

Diagnosis

Nymphomania due to follicular cysts is the diagnosis.

Treatment

Insert a PRID for 12 days – nymphomaniacal behaviour will cease in about 24 h. Oestrus will occur 2–3 days after its withdrawal when the cow should be served. Alternatively GnRH or hCG can be used to cause luteinization of the cysts with cessation of behavioural problems, these will often regress spontaneously after 2–3 weeks. Sometimes it is worthwhile causing premature lysis of these structures with $PGF_{2\alpha}$.

There is some evidence that cystic ovarian disease is inherited and therefore treatment with retention of progeny is questionable. Early treatment is important to prevent injury to the individual cow and others in the herd, and to overcome the problems of disruption of oestrus detection.

ABNORMAL VULVAL DISCHARGE

At many times during the reproductive life of the cow it will be normal for there to be a vulval discharge. At oestrus it will be a clear, elastic mucus; at metoestrus a slightly cloudy and fresh blood-stained mucus; after calving a reddish brown, odourless discharge.

History

Calved 6 weeks ago; dystocia perhaps caused by twins or fetal oversize, followed by placental retention for 6 days (or calving and the periparturient period may have been normal); milk yield slightly below anticipated level (or it may be normal); obvious purulent vulval discharge observed 2 days ago when cow was in oestrus.

Clinical examination

Good health and reasonable bodily condition; soiling of base of tail, tail switch and perineum; not pregnant but uterine horns are of a dissimilar size with oedema of the uterine wall; ovaries are normal with early corpus luteum developing; specular examination shows a copious volume of mucopurulent material pooling in the vagina.

Diagnosis

The diagnosis is leukorrhoea caused by endometritis. It is important to examine the vestibular mucosa for the presence of lesions. If large numbers of animals are involved the possibility of a vaginitis caused by infection with genital infectious bovine rhinotracheitis and *Ureaplasma* species should be considered.

Treatment

Inject $PGF_{2\alpha}$ in 7 days' time, or 3 mg oestradiol benzoate at the time of examination. Intrauterine irrigation with 0.5–1.0 l of physiological saline can be effective. The intrauterine infusion of a broad-spectrum antibiotic (oxytetracycline) at a therapeutic dose rate followed by withdrawal of milk may be considered.

FURTHER READING

ADAS (1984). *Dairy Herd Fertility*. ADAS reference book 259. HMSO, London.
Arthur, G. H., Noakes, D. E. & Pearson, H. (1982). *Veterinary Reproduction and Obstetrics*. Baillière Tindall, London.
Boyd, H. & Noakes, D. E. (1985). *The Individual Infertile Cow*. Number 40. Unit for Veterinary Continuing Education, Royal Veterinary College, London.
Peters, A. R. & Ball, J. J. H. (1987). *Reproduction in Cattle*. Butterworths, London.

CHAPTER 8

Torsion of the Uterus in the Cow

IAN BAKER

INTRODUCTION

Torsion of the uterus in the cow has been defined as the rotation of the uterus on its long axis with twisting of the anterior vagina. It is a common cause of dystocia with a reported incidence of 5–7 %.

The degree of rotation varies, rotation up to 360° being common but rotations to 720° (double twist) are uncommon. The direction of rotation also varies. The anticlockwise revolution is most common, the assessment being made by a vaginal examination.

The torsion usually affects the anterior vagina. This is especially noticeable in torsions of 270° or more. The effect is akin to "putting one's arm up a rifle barrel"!

The majority of uterine torsions occur at the time of parturition. The author has only encountered one torsion prior to parturition (at 8 months' gestation) in 20 years of farm animal practice.

AETIOLOGY

The exact cause of torsion of the uterus in cows is uncertain but the following points may be important:

(1)   The calf is usually larger than average.
(2)   It occurs at late first stage/early second stage of labour.
(3)   The instability of the gravid bovine uterus in its suspension from the pelvis by the broad ligaments.
(4)   Fetal movements during the first stage of labour which result in the repositioning of the calf ready for parturition.
(5)   The age, parity or breed of the cow have no effect on the incidence of the condition.

SIGNS

The main presenting sign is a cow which appears to start calving and progresses no further than the first stage of labour. With a 360° torsion the fetal membranes usually remain intact. Affected cows often show all the unease and mild pain associated with a parturient cow. With torsions of 270° or less it is quite common for the fetal membranes to rupture.

Ventral oedema can occur in cases which have been in labour for 2–3 days.

DIAGNOSIS

With experience, diagnosis is easy on vaginal examination. Where there is a 360° torsion the spiral "rifling" of the anterior vagina is obvious. This effect is less palpable with lower degrees of torsion and a diagnosis depends more on the position of the calf.

The direction of the torsion is not easy to determine. When the torsion occurs anterior to the cervix and the vagina is not involved, the condition presents as a partially dilated cervix which, if one is able to penetrate, then a solid wall of tissue is palpable. These cases are not common and diagnosis can be confirmed by rectal examination.

TREATMENT

MANIPULATION PER VAGINUM

This is most easily achieved in cows that are standing and where the cervix can be entered and the calf reached. A calf's leg is grasped and the calf rocked with sufficient force to correct the torsion.

MANIPULATION BY ROLLING THE COW

The method is used where manipulation per vaginum is not successful or when the torsion is 360° or more. The cow is cast on to its side, usually with a rope using Reuff's method; it should be cast on to the same side as the direction of the torsion. Position the legs and quickly roll the cow over to the other side and then into sternal recumbency. A hand may be held in the vagina during this procedure although it is not necessary except to confirm the diagnosis of the direction of the twist and the success of the treatment. In some cases this rolling procedure has to be repeated for the torsion to be fully corrected. There are refinements to this simple rolling technique such as the use of a board. In my opinion these refinements are not necessary. However, details of them can be found in the references.

SURGICAL CORRECTION

If the torsion is irreducible by manipulation then it can be reduced via a laparotomy. In effect this means delivering the fetus by caesarean section. It is advisable to attempt to reduce the torsion before incising the uterus since after removing the fetus and then correcting the torsion the uterine wound can end up in a position where it is difficult to repair. Care must also be taken when handling such a uterus as it is often very oedematous and liable to rupture.

COMPLICATIONS

The following complications may arise:

(1)   Incomplete dilation of the cervis is common. If possible deliver the fetus at once. If the cervix will not allow this then some relaxation may occur in 30–60 min. The use of specific smooth muscle relaxants (such as dimophebumine [Monzaldon] or clenbuterol; [Planipart, Boehringer Ingelheim]) may help this relaxation. If the calf is alive it should be delivered as soon as possible as early placental separation and fetal death can occur with a torsion of the uterus. If the cervix fails to dilate then the calf must be delivered by caesarian section.
(2)   Uterine rupture. The uterus may rupture, this can occur during delivery of the calf through a poorly dilated cervix. The rupture is usually transverse and occurs just cranial to the cervix.
(3)   Peritonitis can occur following the correction of a torsion. All cases should receive 5 days' broad-spectrum antibiotic therapy as a routine.
(4)   Post-parturient metritis is a common sequel, and should be treated in the normal manner.

FURTHER READING

Arthur, G. H., Noakes, D. E. & Pearson, H. (1982). *Veterinary Reproduction and Obstetrics*, 5th edn., Baillière Tindall, London.
Duncanson, G. R. (1984). *Proceedings British Cattle Veterinary Association*, p. 133. Available from Pearson, H. (1971). *Veterinary Record* **89**, 597.
Roberts, S. J. (1956). *Veterinary Obstetrics and General Diseases*. Ithaca, New York.

CHAPTER 9

Prolapse of the Uterus in the Cow

BOB PLENDERLEITH

INTRODUCTION

Prolapse of the uterus in the cow usually occurs immediately after or within a few hours of parturition.

In practice, the condition is recorded as occurring in 0.5 % of all assisted calvings and in 0.3 % of all parturitions. Prolapse is considered to occur as a result of atony of the myometrium of the uterus and expansion of the broad ligaments, along with relaxation of the perineal and perivaginal tissues. There are a number of predisposing factors, which are listed in Table 9.1.

CORRECTION OF THE PROLAPSE

The ease of correction will depend on many complicating factors including the duration of the prolapse, its size and whether the animal is recumbent or has concurrent disease.

Many operators, especially with heifers, will replace the prolapse in the standing animal with or without the use of epidural (extradural) anaesthetic. If any difficulty is encountered the animal should be cast using Reuff's method and replacement undertaken as follows (Fig. 9.1).

Table 9.1 Predisposing factors to prolapse of the uterus.

Hypocalcaemia   This is an important factor in the dairy cow. In the beef cow, low calcium and low calcium–phosphorus ratios have been recorded.

Retained placenta   This may stimulate excessive contractions

Oversized fetus   More cases are occurring in beef cows and this is a possible factor associated with traction. The presence of larger hips and hindquarters in "exotic" breeds is possibly important because a contracting uterus will cling more readily to the fetus

Traction   The condition is more common in association with traction. Too rapid fetal extraction or expulsion may be important. The misuse of calving machines is particularly a problem on farms where labour is short

Prolonged dystocia   This can arise as a result of hypocalcaemia, an oversized fetus and traction. Exhaustion may also be a contributing factor

Chronic disease   Occasionally a number of cases occur within one beef herd when the cows are in poor condition during malnutrition or specific diseases (e.g. parasitism, copper deficiency, etc.)

Paresis   This can occur as a result of chronic disease or injury following calving. Obturator or sciatic paralysis can be complicating factors

The cow is rolled on to one side and the leg on the opposite side is pulled straight back. The cow is then rolled to the opposite side and the process repeated. The animal is then pushed to lie on its abdomen with both hindlegs pulled straight out behind and the prolapse positioned between its legs. An extra person, if available, should sit astride the cow, facing posteriorly and holding the tail straight up.

After first cleansing and disinfecting the uterus, it is then either placed on a board or a bale covered by a clean sheet, held in a sheet by two assistants or held by the operator himself, depending on personal choice. In the majority of cases the uterus is easily replaced by working initially from the vaginal end and finally by gentle pressure. Care must be taken to make sure the uterine horns are completely everted.

The animal is returned to a comfortable sitting position and the vagina sutured with deep mattress sutures or with a Brahner's buried purse string suture using 0.25 in tape. Many operators feel that suturing is unnecessary if the prolapse has been properly returned, but it seems a logical precaution to take if the condition is not to recur.

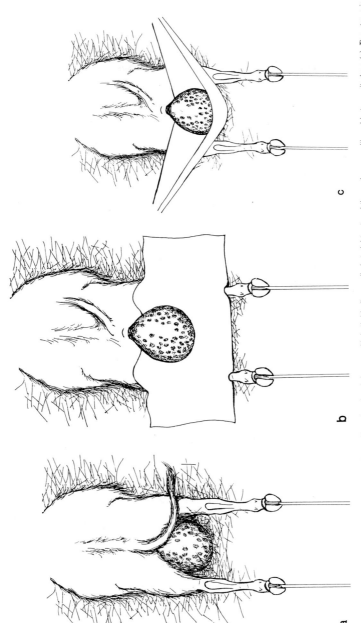

Fig. 9.1 Sequence of events during which the cow is positioned on its abdomen, with both hindlegs pulled straight out and the prolapse positioned between its legs (a). The uterus is then placed on a bale covered by a clean sheet (b) or held in a sheet by two assistants or the operator (c).

The writer has not found it necessary to use an epidural anaesthetic, but acknowledges that it might help by suspending defecation during return of the prolapse and by postponing straining.

If the prolapse is very enlarged the use of oxytocin either by intramuscular (50 iu), intravenous (10 iu) or intrauterine (50 iu) routes may be useful. Bathing with hypertonic saline solution is helpful.

The β-adrenergic drug clenbuterol hydrochloride has been recommended for use in this condition. It should not be used with corticosteroids or atropine, or in association with epidural or general anaesthesia, and it is antagonistic to the effects of prostaglandin $F_{2\alpha}$ and oxytocin.

Routine antibiotic cover should be given for 3–4 days following correction of the prolapse.

Table 9.2 Complications in prolapse of the uterus.

Hypocalcaemia Treatment of affected cows should be carried out where possible before replacement, in case regurgitation and aspiration of ruminal contents occur during the handling of the cow, or in case it succumbs to the hypocalcaemia

Haemorrhage This may lead to hypovolaemic shock and haemoconcentration and should be arrested and the lesion sutured. Two litres of citrated blood may be useful. Injection of iron (1000–2000 mg) plus 3000 μg of hydroxocobalamin is recommended. A case of death due to haemorrhage into the abdomen from ovarian vessels has been encountered recently in an apparently uncomplicated replacement

Metritis

Peritonitis

Toxaemia/septicaemia

Fractures

Paresis

Necrosis Degrees of necrosis and gangrene on long standing cases can be present

Rupture Prolapse of intestine or bladder

COMPLICATIONS

A number of complications can arise and these are listed in Table 9.2. In cases of necrosis, gangrene or severe rupture, amputation of the uterus may be indicated. If so, first ascertain, by incision if necessary, whether any intestine or the bladder is enclosed within the prolapse; reduce if present. Then ligate, with two large sutures, the vagina just posterior to the cervix, ensuring the lateral vaginal arteries are included. Ligate the middle uterine and uterovarian arteries on both sides, incise and remove.

In spite of the many possible complicating factors, the prognosis for correction of the prolapsed uterus is usually good with an expected recovery rate of 85 %. The recurrence at subsequent parturitions or the effect on fertility do not seem to have been carefully recorded.

Disease and Medical Problems

CHAPTER 10

Amputation of the Bovine Digit

IAN BAKER

PREPARATION

Indications for amputation of the bovine digit are summarized in Table 10.1. According to preference, amputation of the bovine digit can be performed with the animal recumbent or standing, with or without the affected limb lifted. The author prefers to have the patient standing with the affected limb lifted – a specially designed "foot crush" (e.g. Woppa Box) is very useful for this purpose.

Sedation using an intramuscular injection of xylazine (Rompun; Bayer) 5–30 mg/100 kg bodyweight is necessary when the operation is performed on a recumbent animal but is usually unnecessary when it is performed on the standing animal.

The whole of the leg below the hock or carpus is thoroughly cleansed using a surgical scrub. The materials required are listed in Table 10.2 and the anatomy of the digit is shown in Fig. 10.1. A suitable case for amputation is shown in Fig. 10.2.

Table 10.1 Indications for amputation of the digit.

Traumatic injury to hoof

Severe penetrations of the sole

Sepsis and septic arthritis of the first (distal) interphalangeal joint

Septic tenosynovitis of the deep flexor tendon

Osteomyelitis of the third phalanx

TECHNIQUE

A tourniquet is applied to the mid-tarsal/mid-carpal region or above the hock. In a "foot crush" the loop used for lifting the leg makes an ideal tourniquet on the hindlimb. The tourniquet is applied for the duration of the operation.

Local anaesthesia is induced with 30 ml of a 2 % solution of lignocaine hydrochloride without adrenalin injected into a convenient superficial vein (Edwards, 1981). When anaesthesia

Table 10.2 Materials required.

Syringes 5 ml, 20 ml, 30 ml

Needles 25×0.9 mm (20 gauge $\times$ 1 in) and 1.2×40 mm (18 gauge $\times$ 1.5 in)

Veterinary scrub (Pevidine; Berk Pharmaceuticals)

Xylazine (Rompun; Bayer)

Local anaesthetic (2 % lignocaine hydrochloride)

Scalpel

1 m embryotomy wire

Embryotomy wire holders

Antibiotics – long-acting preparations such as penicillin or oxytetracycline

Broad-spectrum antibiotic powder (Aureomycin topical powder; Cyanamid)

Dry dressings

Bandages

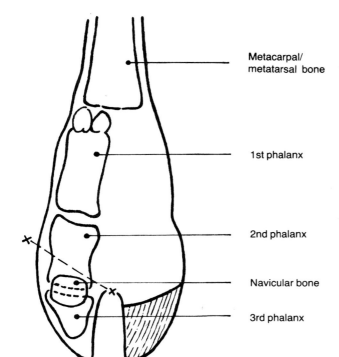

Metacarpal/
metatarsal bone

1st phalanx

2nd phalanx

Navicular bone

3rd phalanx

Fig. 10.1
Anatomy of the
bovine digit.

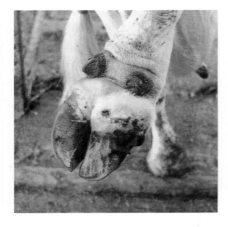

Fig. 10.2
A suitable case for amputation – an infected lateral
claw of the right hindlimb.

is complete a deep incision is made in the interdigital space close to the affected digit and along its whole length.

The embryotomy wire (Fig. 10.3) is introduced into this incision and the claw amputated by sawing through the lower third of the second phalanx. This is achieved by sawing rapidly at an oblique angle so that the cut emerges 2–3 cm above the coronary band on the abaxial surface. The stump is examined for any signs of necrosis or infection which are curretted away. Any protruding interdigital fat is also removed.

The wound is dressed with a broad-spectrum antibiotic powder (e.g. Aureomycin topical powder; Cyanamid), a dry dressing applied (Melolin; Smith & Nephew) and a gauze pad is placed over this and held in place using a conforming bandage (Crinx; Smith & Nephew). A pressure bandage is applied to the lower third of the leg and the tourniquet released. Prophylactic long-acting antibiotic injection is given, usually procaine/benethamine penicillin (Propen; Glaxo) or oxytetracycline (Terramycin LA; Pfizer).

The pressure bandage is removed after 3–6 days by which time the stump is covered in granulation tissue (Fig. 10.4). The wound is redressed without the pressure bandage.

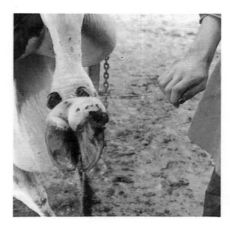

Fig. 10.3
Positioning of embryotomy wire before amputation of the claw.

POSTOPERATIVE CARE

The animal should be housed on a flat surface such as concrete. Rough areas such as straw yards or rutted fields are likely to touch the healing stump and cause pain.

The owner should be instructed to remove the dressing after 14 days and then keep the whole area as clean as possible. Complete healing should take between 4 and 6 weeks.

COMPLICATIONS

Haemorrhage is usually well controlled by the tourniquet but it does occur occasionally. It is difficult to pick up and ligate the bleeding vessels and the haemorrhage is best controlled by applying a pressure bandage.

It is important to use non-adherent dressings on the wound, otherwise when they are removed a large part of the granulation tissue will also come away causing the wound to bleed.

Infection caused by inadequate removal of septic tissue at the time of the operation and postoperative abscessation may occur, and may even spread to include the other digit.

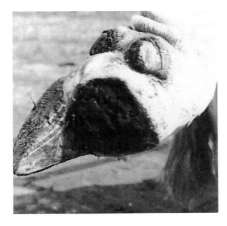

Fig. 10.4
Stump 4 days after amputation.

Table 10.3 Advantages and disadvantages of digit removal.

Advantages	Disadvantages
Relief of pain	A failure to return to normality if the wrong case is selected for amputation
Removal of a septic focus allowing good drainage	
Relatively rapid return to soundness with corresponding increase in body condition and milk yield	A persistent poor gait in some animals
The technique is simple	

DISCUSSION

The advantages and disadvantages of amputation are listed in Table 10.3. Some veterinarians recommend the exarticulation of the second phalanx because it is said that the remaining proximal part of the second phalanx undergoes necrosis and impairs healing. In the author's experience this seldom happens, or at least healing is not impaired, so this simpler method is preferred.

REFERENCES AND FURTHER READING

Edwards, G. B. (1981). *Veterinary Record* Supplement. *In Practice* **6**(3), 13.
Greenough, P. R., MacCallum, F. J. & Weaver, A. D. (1981). *Lameness in Cattle,* 3nd edn. John Wright Scientechnica, Bristol.
Weaver, A. D. (1986). *Bovine Surgery and Lameness.* Blackwell Scientific Publications, Oxford.

CHAPTER 11

Nitrate/Nitrite Poisoning in Cattle

T. O. JONES

INTRODUCTION

In the public mind, there is an association between the use of artificial nitrogenous fertilizers in agriculture and an increased incidence of illness caused by nitrogen compounds, mainly via mains water. Although this view must be respected and the situation kept under review, poisoning in humans by nitrates in water appears uncommon. The last reported UK death of a baby from nitrate poisoning occurred in 1950 and the last confirmed non-fatal case in 1972. The incidence of human stomach cancer, once claimed to be related to consumption of high-nitrate content water has decreased significantly in the past 20 years. Well water supplies to farms and country houses are much more likely to contain dangerously high nitrate levels than is mains water. Food is the main human dietary source of nitrate. In cattle, almost all the recorded cases of nitrate poisoning have been caused by the consumption of plant material of high nitrate content. The condition is probably uncommon in the UK.

AETIOLOGY

Nitrates are found commonly in nature. While large amounts cause gastroenteritis, they are relatively non-toxic but may be converted to lethal nitrite by a number of common species of bacteria including *Clostridia* and *Enterobacteria*. In single-stomached animals, conversion occurs mainly in the caecum and colon. In such animals, dietary nitrate is absorbed from the small intestine and excreted via the kidneys before reaching the caecum. In contrast, rapid conversion of nitrate to nitrite can occur in the rumen. Where there is adequate carbohydrate in the ration, much of the nitrate may be converted to ammonia.

All mammals are susceptible to the potential toxic effects of preformed nitrites in the diet. Conversion of nitrate to nitrite may occur in oat hay in a stack, particularly if it is wet and hot or damp for some time before feeding. Slow cooking of mangels may convert nitrate to nitrite. There is one report of monensin dietary supplementation precipitating nitrite poisoning in cattle, presumably as a result of interference with rumen microflora. Common sources of nitrate and nitrite are shown in Table 11.1.

EPIDEMIOLOGY

Nitrate is absorbed from the soil by plants and eventually converted into plant protein. When excess accumulation of nitrate occurs, the plant may be toxic to ruminants. Factors encouraging accumulation of nitrate by plants are listed in Table 11.2.

Under extensive grazing conditions abroad, nitrate poisoning is seen in animals in poor condition grazing unfertilized pasture after drought. There have been serious problems in Holland associated with over-application of inorganic nitrogenous fertilizer to land which had already received adequate manure. In England, cases have been described in association with excess application to pasture of sewage sludge and farmyard manure. In Scotland the condition was typically seen in animals grazing kale, on overcast cold November days

Table 11.1 Common sources of nitrate.

Crops: Oat hay, immature green oats, barley, wheat and rye hay. Barley straw, Sudan grass, maize, sorghum (hybrid varieties in particular). Rye grass, brassicae, lettuce (horticultural surplus)

Organic fertilizer

Inorganic fertilizer

Water contaminated with fertilizer – organic and inorganic

Nitrate accumulating weeds

Industrial pollution of water (cheese, meat preserving and rubber curing)

Certain explosives

Silage preservatives

Disinfectant for water pipes (used by water authorities)

Table 11.2 Factors associated with accumulation of nitrates in growing plants.

Excessive nitrate in soil due to:
  Heavy application of animal slurry or sewage
  Heavy application of inorganic nitrogenous fertilizer, especially during drought
  High temperature encouraging nitrification by soil bacteria
  Drought – absence of leaching

Molybdenum deficiency and/or tungsten excess

Damage to plants by herbicides and insects

Species of plant

Insufficient sunlight – reduced photosynthesis

Possibly reduced ambient temperature

and thought to be partly caused by suboptimal photosynthesis. In the USA and Australia, particularly, the condition is caused by consumption of weed species which accumulate nitrate.

Although water in ditches and ponds in the UK may have naturally high nitrate content, no case of nitrate poisoning from this source has been reported. However, the author has investigated deaths of dairy cows from acute nitrate poisoning caused by consumption of water containing 1496 mg/l nitrite and 792 mg/l nitrate, as a result of pollution from a factory processing rubber.

Deaths following the consumption of ammonium nitrate fertilizer are not always due to nitrate poisoning. Death may be related either to ammonium poisoning or to some other unknown toxic mechanism.

PATHOGENESIS

Nitrite causes vasodilation and conversion of haemoglobin into non-oxygen carrying methaemoglobin. Signs of disease due to the anaemic anoxia occur in cattle when 20 % of haemoglobin has been converted to methaemoglobin and death occurs when 60–80 % has been converted. In cattle and sheep, maximum methaemoglobinaemia occurs about 5 h after ingestion of nitrate-rich vegetation (Fig. 11.1). Young cattle may be more susceptible. Horses may show signs of distress when only 5 % of methaemoglobin is present. Vasodilation prior to formation of detectable levels of methaemoglobin has been claimed to cause sudden death in a horse and there is one report of a similar syndrome in cattle.

CLINICAL SIGNS AND POST-MORTEM FINDINGS

Acute nitrate/nitrite poisoning presents dramatic disease signs (Table 11.3). Figure 11.1 demonstrates the colour changes seen in vaginal mucous membranes associated with known levels of methaemoglobin. Abortion may occur as a sequel to acute sublethal nitrate/nitrite poisoning in cattle. However, claims that excess nitrate ingestion can cause abortion in livestock without other signs of poisoning being exhibited have not been substantiated experimentally. In Holland, a high incidence of mummified fetuses has been recorded in the autumn following non-fatal nitrate toxicity during the summer. Stillbirths have been reproduced experimentally by intravenous injection of nitrite at parturition but only after appreciable quantities of methaemoglobin have been formed.

Field reports and experimental studies with laboratory

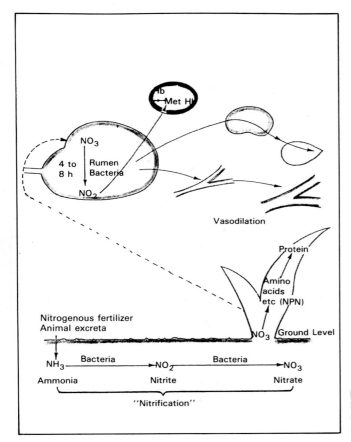

Fig. 11.1
Nitrogen cycle and
nitrate/nitrite
poisoning in cattle.

animals have incriminated chronic sublethal nitrate poisoning as a causal or contributing factor in a variety of conditions, including reduced growth and production, abortion and interference with both iodine and vitamin A metabolism. Attempts to substantiate these reports have produced varied and often contradictory results. Compensatory erythropoietic responses with raised haemoglobin concentrations, PCVs and increased blood volume, may occur in pregnant heifers receiving excess nitrate for long periods. In one experiment, heifers receiving high nitrate content rations grew more rapidly than controls. Could it be that factors in the diet, in addition to nitrate have been involved in some field cases?

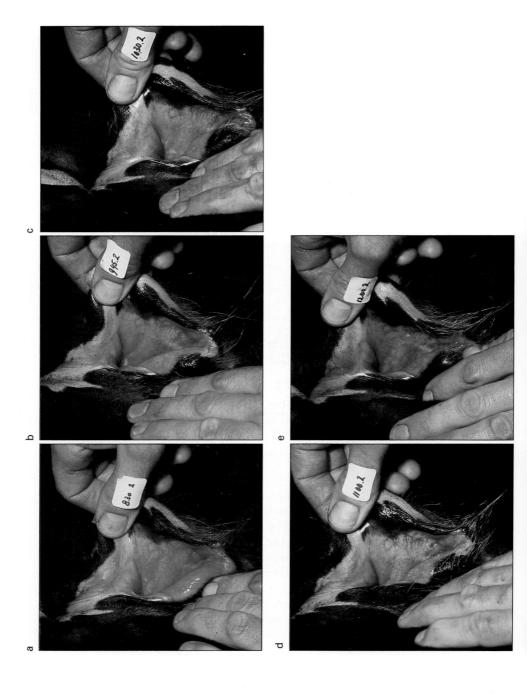

Table 11.3 Signs of nitrate/nitrite poisoning in cattle.

Very rapid breathing

Dyspnoea with gasping

Fast jugular pulse (up to 200/min)

Mucous membranes brown/grey

Abdominal pain with diarrhoea

Muscle tremor, weakness, staggering gait, severe cyanosis followed by blanching of mucosa

Normal/subnormal temperature

Frequent urination and dripping of urine

Collapse, convulsions and death within 30 min of the first signs of disease

Abortion may be a sequel to non-fatal disease

In one reported incident cardiac and circulatory failure without other signs was the most common syndrome

For example, it is known that dietary amines cause enteritis. In the case of industrial pollution previously mentioned, pregnant dairy cows consumed water containing very high levels of nitrite and nitrate for several weeks and cows died of poisoning but there was no abortion.

The principal post-mortem findings in ruminants are chocolate brown discoloration of blood and tissues, poor clotting of blood, cardiac haemorrhage and pulmonary congestion. In my experience, the urinary bladder is tightly contracted. After prolonged decomposition, blood may appear pink due to the formation of red nitric oxide haemoglobin.

DIAGNOSIS

In situations where nitrate/nitrite poisoning is a possibility the occurrence of characteristic clinical signs and the presence of brown blood is sufficient evidence for a tentative diagnosis. Several other disease entities show similar clinical signs and post-mortem findings (Table 11.4).

The diphenylamine test is used to detect nitrate/nitrite in clear body fluids. Aqueous humour, CSF, serum and urine are most suitable for testing. The diphenylamine test is not specific for nitrate/nitrite. A variety of cations not normally found in the body are capable of giving positive reactions. It will detect 1 ppm NO_2 and 10 ppm NO_3. In the author's experience, a strong positive result is needed to confirm a diagnosis. Commercial test strips for nitrate and nitrite testing are available.

The detection of methaemoglobin is not specific for nitrate poisoning, although it is stated to be only likely to be present in large quantities in one other condition, sodium chlorate poisoning. In the author's experience, appreciable quantities may be found terminally in chronic copper poisoning. Methaemoglobin is unstable and estimations should be carried out immediately specimens are collected. If fresh, preferably heparinized, blood samples are lysed in nine volumes of distilled water, the methaemoglobin remains stable. Blood samples from animals *in extremis* will appear obviously brown to the sampler.

Other specimens for laboratory examination should include ingesta and suspected plants/soil/water. The addition of chloroform or formalin to prevent bacterial conversion of nitrates is advisable. Deep freezing is also an acceptable method of preservation.

Nitrate/nitrite estimation of diet is usually indicated. It is stated that concentrations of dietary nitrate greater than 1 %

Table 11.4 Differential diagnosis of acute nitrate/nitrite poisoning in cattle.

Sodium chlorate poisoning

Silo gases (NO, NO_2, N_2O_4) poisoning

Acute kale poisoning (blood anaemic)

Cyanide poisoning (blood cherry red)

Carbon dioxide poisoning (blood dark blue)

Carbon monoxide poisoning (blood bright red)

Chronic copper poisoning crisis (blood brown)

Note: Dark blood, not brown, may be found in the terminal stages of a variety of conditions.

---

dry matter are necessary to cause poisoning. Figure 11.3 demonstrates the relationship between the nitrate level in roughage, dry matter intake and methaemoglobin levels achieved in blood. The diphenylamine test (Table 11.5) has been used on plant tissue. An intense blue colour within 10 s indicates a concentration of greater than 1 % nitrate. This is best used as a screening test. High levels of nitrate may be localized in a field – single hay bales have been found to contain lethal nitrate levels whereas other bales from the same field were safe. Nitrate levels in plants may vary during the course of the day, being higher in the early morning. A high non-protein nitrogen (NPN) value in silage does not necessarily mean that its nitrate content is high.

OTHER TOXIC DERIVATIVES

Nitrosamines (*N*-nitroso compounds) are chemical derivatives of nitrite which are toxic and can be carcinogenic. They are commonly found in silage and at least 100 different nitrosamine compounds are capable of producing various tumours in laboratory animals. A nitrosamine found in plant food has been proven to cause oesophageal cancer in the Bantu. Evidence linking consumption of high nitrate content water

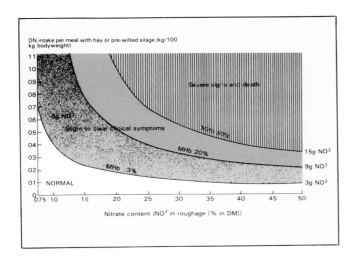

Fig. 11.3
The nitrate content and the dry matter intake of preserved grass in relation to the formation of methaemoglobin (Geurink *et al.*, 1982).

Table 11.5 The diphenylamine test.

Principle

Nitrate and nitrite anions oxidize diphenylamine or its oxidation product diphenylbenzidine in concentrated sulphuric acid to an intensely blue quinoidal compound. Bromides, iodates, chlorates, selenites, molybdates, iron, antimony and peroxides also give a positive reaction if the concentration is high enough. Under normal circumstances it is unlikely that these substances would interfere. Serum, urine, thoracic, peritoneal or pericardial fluids, bile or foetal bile may be tested. Deeply coloured specimens are unsuitable for this test.

Reagent

(1) 0.5 % (29.55 mmol/l) diphenylamine in 80 % (800 ml/l) sulphuric acid. Add 80 ml of concentrated sulphuric acid carefully to a cooled beaker containing 0.5 g (2.955 mmol) of the reagent and 20 ml of water, stir carefully and cool.
(2) Dilute the stock reagent 5 ml to 40 ml with concentrated sulphuric acid.

Procedure

Put a drop of the fluid to be tested on a white tile. Add three drops of the diluted reagent. An immediate intense blue colour indicates the presence of nitrate or nitrite.

Reference

Householder, G. T., Dollahite, J. M. & Hulse, R. (1966) *Journal of the American Veterinary Medical Association* **148**, 662.

with human stomach cancer has been presented in the UK but more extensive studies have refuted this.

Herring meal containing high levels of dimethylnitrosamine was responsible for extensive centrilobular liver necrosis, fibrosis and death of cattle, sheep, chicks, mink and foxes in Norway. Large quantities of sodium nitrite had been added to the herring meal during processing. Nitrites are no longer used as a preservative in fishmeal in the UK.

THERAPY

Methylene blue converts methaemoglobin to haemoglobin. A recommended regime of therapy is the administration of a vasoconstrictor such as adrenalin or etamiphylline camsylate intravenously, followed by 1–2 mg/kg bodyweight methylene blue administered intravenously as a 1 % solution.

There are reports of successful therapy using a vasoconstrictor alone, but the amount of nitrate which had been consumed is not recorded. Paradoxically, high doses of methylene blue cause methaemoglobinaemia in some species. However, this does not appear to occur in cattle and sheep, and a high dose rate of 20 mg/kg body weight is recommended by some workers. The half-life of methylene blue in tissues is about 2 h, and repetition of treatment may be necessary at 6–8 h intervals. Oral administration of formalin or antibiotics to destroy the rumen flora which convert nitrate to nitrite may also be indicated.

PROPHYLAXIS AND CONTROL

Nitrate/nitrite poisoning in cattle from forages is so uncommon in the UK that widespread publicity on prophylaxis is probably not justified.

The condition is more common in Holland, and where silage analysis shows a crude protein value of 20 % or more, the farmer is routinely warned of the danger of nitrate poisoning and recommended to have a nitrate estimation carried out on his silage. Routine examination at milking time of cows' vaginal mucous membranes for bown/grey discoloration is also recommended.

Cattle likely to be exposed to excess nitrate should receive adequate dietary carbohydrate.

High nitrate content grass is more dangerous after wilting and the problem of poisoning is more severe in European countries where grass is cut and wilted before being fed to housed cows. In Poland, routine incorporation of wolfram (tungsten) in the diet as prophylaxis for nitrate poisoning has been seriously considered.

A large number of nitrate accumulating plants (mostly weeds) have been described abroad but not in the UK. One subject which should receive attention is the nitrate content of new grass and other feeding crop varieties. The introduction of hybrid sorghums in America was followed by large scale outbreaks of nitrate poisoning as these accumulated nitrate in certain situations.

REFERENCES AND FURTHER READING

Kemp, I. A., Geurink, J. H., Haalstra, R. T. & Malestein, I. A. (1976). *Dutch Nitrogenous Fertiliser Review* **19**, 40–48.
Geurink, J. H., Malestein, A., Kemp, A., Korzeniowsky, A. & van't Klooster, A. Th. (1982). *Netherlands Journal of Agricultural Science* **30**, 105–113.

CHAPTER 12

Magnesium and Milk Fever

JIM KELLY

INTRODUCTION

As the milk yield of dairy cows in the UK has increased by 30 % over the past 20 years, so the overall incidence of milk fever has risen from around 3 % to over 7 % in newly calved cows. Individual farms can have an incidence of between 60 and 70 % during certain periods of the year. Just as the incidence can vary from farm to farm and from year to year, it can vary with the age of the cow and with breed. Jersey cows, for example, are more susceptible to milk fever, probably because of their high milk production in relation to their body size.

Although the exact mechanisms involved are not completely understood it has been demonstrated frequently that the management and nutrition of the cow during the dry period can have a strong influence on the susceptibility of individual animals to the condition.

The well-recognized clinical signs are essentially caused by a rapid decrease in the concentration of calcium in the blood which occurs close to parturition. The basic reason for the hypocalcaemia is the inability of some cows to match their rapidly increasing requirements for calcium for milk secretion by absorbing sufficient calcium from their gut or by mobilizing calcium from their own skeleton. Magnesium has been shown to play an important role in influencing the absorption of calcium from the intestine and the mobilization of calcium from bone. Autumn blood tests have demonstrated that 20–30 % of dry cows had blood magnesium concentrations less than 0.78 mmol/l.

AETIOLOGY

The minimum calcium requirements shown in Fig. 12.1 have been estimated by assuming that 68 % of the calcium in the diet is absorbed from the intestine. Information is imprecise as to what proportion of dietary calcium can be absorbed. It is more likely that ruminants absorb calcium according to bodily need, and the role is increased by the action of 1,25 dihydroxy vitamin D_3.

Within a few hours of calving the demand for calcium may have doubled. To maintain a normal concentration of calcium in blood either the absorption of calcium from the gut must be increased rapidly or calcium must be mobilized from the skeleton (Fig. 12.2). Normally both these processes occur together but if they fail to meet the demand, hypocalcaemia occurs and, as it becomes more profound, the clinical symptoms of milk fever develop.

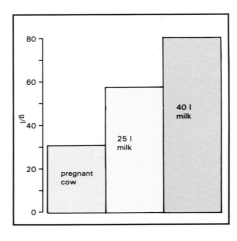

Fig. 12.1
Dietary calcium requirements for dry and lactating cows.

When calcium levels in the blood fall the parathyroid gland is stimulated to release parathyroid hormone (PTH) which acts on the bones releasing calcium and phosphorus. Its other, and probably more important, role is the stimulation of the production of the hydroxylase enzyme in the kidney which is responsible for the second of two hydroxylation steps which convert vitamin D to its active hormonal form, 1,25 dihydroxy vitamin D_3. This hormone assists in stimulating the absorption of calcium from the gut and the mobilization of calcium from the bone. The speed and extent of the response to PTH and 1,25 dihydroxy vitamin D_3 is governed by several factors:

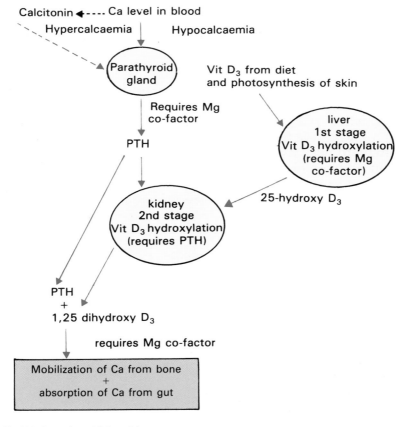

Fig. 12.2 System for mobilizing calcium.

(1) *Age*. Older cows may be slower to respond by mobilizing calcium from bone and this, in addition to the tendency for milk yield to increase with age, may partly explain why older cows are more susceptible to milk fever.

(2) *Oestrogens*, which increase at calving, tend to inhibit calcium mobilization. Normal cyclical increases in oestrogen during lactation have been associated with clinical signs of milk fever occurring several weeks after calving. During oestrus feed intake is frequently reduced and this may also result in a reduction of available calcium.

(3) *Hypomagnesaemia*. This may interfere with release of PTH; hydroxylation of vitamin D in liver; and mobilization of calcium from bones and absorption of calcium from the gut.

CLINICAL SIGNS

The classical symptoms of milk fever are well recognized. In the first stage the cow becomes dull and lethargic and loses her appetite. She is afebrile and the ears may be cold to the touch. There may be an initial period of hypersensitivity and tetany with head shaking and teeth grinding. Stiffness of legs becomes apparent and typical straight hocks and "paddling" from one foot to the other may be seen. As hypocalcaemia becomes more severe the cow becomes recumbent (Fig. 12.3). At first the cow is in sternal recumbency with a lateral kink in the neck and the head turned into the flank. Pulse rate increases (70–80/min). The pupils dilate with a reduced pupillary light reflex. Ruminal stasis develops and the cow

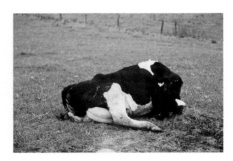

Fig. 12.3
Recumbent cow with milk fever.

does not urinate or defecate. Finally, the cow lies on her side and becomes comatose. Pulse rate is high (120/min) when laterally recumbent and very weak. Tympany of the rumen or inhalation of regurgitated rumen contents may cause respiratory failure.

If hypocalcaemia occurs before calving, uterine inertia may occur. If calving does occur, severe hypocalcaemia may result in prolapse of uterus. Normally the severity of symptoms relate to the severity of hypocalcaemia.

At calving blood calcium levels fall. The normal range is 2.2–2.6 mmol/l. Clinical signs appear at levels below 1.5 mmol/l. These may go as low as 0.25 mg/l. Blood phosphorus levels fall at calving. Normal range is 1.4–2.5 mmol/l. In milk fever it is below 1 mmol/l. Magnesium level in blood normally goes up at calving. If it goes down hypomagnesaemia has a modifying effect on the normal syndrome. Tetany and hyperaesthesia persist beyond the first stage. There may be considerable excitement with typical tetanic convulsions.

It is important to note that low blood magnesium levels in dry cows may result in classical milk fever, for the reasons described above, without clinical signs of hypomagnesaemia.

DIFFERENTIAL DIAGNOSIS

Several conditions can be confused with milk fever (Table 12.1). Some of these develop as sequelae to milk fever. The most practical confirmation of diagnosis is response to treatment.

TREATMENT

Treatment is most effective when given as soon as clinical signs are observed. The best treatment is normally 8–12 g calcium contained in 400 ml of a 40 % solution of calcium borogluconate administered intravenously. Many advocate the inclusion of phosphorus and magnesium, as well as calcium, in the solution, but unless hypomagnesaemia is suspected there is little evidence to suggest that response is any better

Table 12.1 Conditions that can be confused with milk fever.

Disease	Susceptible animals	Clinical signs	Biochemical assessment
Milk fever	Mature cows, especially Channel Island breeds. Most common within 48 h of calving	Early excitement followed by depression and coma. Dilated pupil, weak pulse, cessation of ruminal movement. No defecation	Hypocalcaemia below 1.5 mmol/l. Hypophosphataemia below 1 mmol/l. Magnesium levels may be raised.
Hypomagnesaemia	Any age or stage of lactation. Cows grazing spring or autumn grass more at risk	Excitement and hypersensitivity, tetanic convulsions, loud heart sounds, increased respiratory rates	Low serum magnesium – below 0.8 mmol/l.
Severe toxaemia	Sporadic – may be result of mastitis, metritis or peritonitis. Affects any age of cow	Recumbency, depression, hypothermia, gut statis. Increased heart rate (over 100/min). Grunting. Diarrhoea common	Serum calcium may be slightly reduced; often profound leucopenia

Condition	History/predisposing factors	Demeanour	Biochemistry
Obturator paralysis	Most frequently heifers or young cows. May follow prolonged calving or excessive traction	Bright, alert, eat, drink, defecate, attempt to rise	Calcium, phosphate and magnesium normal CPK may be raised
Injury or fracture of limb	Any age of animal at any stage of lactation. May be sequela to milk fever. Slippery floor increases risk	As for obturator paralysis	Increase in CPK or SGOT depending on extent of muscle damage
Downer cow	Often sequela to milk fever if treatment delayed or nursing poor. May follow overdosing with calcium	Moderately bright except for non-alert downers	Variable – may be hypophosphataemia, low glucose, high ketones. Increased CPK or SGOT
Fatty liver syndrome	Cows recently calved (1–2 weeks). Condition score 3.5 +. May be triggered off by milk fever	Dull depressed. May grunt or moan. No response to treatment	Increase in serum CPK, SGOT, fatty acids, betahydroxybutyrate, bilirubin; decrease in cholesterol, albumen, magnesium

than with calcium alone. If blood sampling has demonstrated that hypophosphataemia is a problem, especially in relapsed cases, then phosphorus in the solution is indicated.

Excessive quantities of calcium, especially when dose is repeated by frequent subcutaneous injection, may dampen the homeostatic responses and result in relapse or recurrence of symptoms. Good nursing and management are necessary if sequelae such as "downer cow" syndrome are to be voided. The calf should be removed and milking restricted.

PREVENTION

Stimulation of the release of PTH and formation of 1,25 dihydroxy vitamin D with resultant increased absorption of calcium from the gut or mobilization from the bone all takes time – at least 24 h. The timing of preventive procedures is therefore important.

DIETARY MANIPULATION

(1)   Avoid high concentration of calcium in the diet during the dry period. This is difficult in practice as most forages, including grass, have a relatively high calcium content. Clover, lucerne, beet pulp and kale have a particularly high calcium content. Pregnant cows require 20–25 g calcium so the diet should contain no more than 50 g calcium. Restrict pasture and feed low-calcium cereals or concentrates during dry period. Supplementation of the diet with phosphate, e.g. monosodium phosphate, is indicated if hypophosphataemia is identified. Opinion differs as to the merit of feeding high-phosphate diets to dry cows. If calcium levels are high they may be contraindicated. The Ca : P ratio does not seem to be so important in ruminants especially when vitamin D status is kept high.
(2)   Drenching with solution of calcium chloride (100–150 g/day for 3 days after calving) can be successful especially if used following a low-calcium diet in the dry period.

(3) Avoid heavy "steaming up". Milking cow concentrate is high in calcium.

(4) Avoid cows being too fat at calving (condition score 3 at most). Fat cows have poor appetites after calving. Mobilization of body fat before calving may cause hypomagnesaemia.

(5) It can be notoriously difficult to raise magnesium levels of dry cows on wet pastures. The absorption of magnesium decreases as potassium content of diet increases; therefore avoid heavy use of nitrogen and potassium. In grazing cows 33 % of magnesium may be absorbed from grass, but this may drop to 20 % from grass grown in highly fertilized areas.

SOURCES OF MAGNESIUM

(1) *Calcined magnesite* in cereal or concentrate (60 g/day) may be most reliable way of ensuring regular supply of magnesium.

(2) *Drinking water.* The addition of magnesium acetate or magnesium chloride can be effective but this method depends on other sources of water being eliminated. This can be difficult in a wet season.

(3) *Pasture dressing.* Calcined magnesite or magnesium lime-stone – variable uptake and availability in wet weather.

(4) *Magnesium licks* or "free access" minerals may not provide sufficient magnesium and intake is not controlled. If this method is used sufficient access points must be provided.

(5) *Magnesium bullets* should be considered where more traditional methods have proved impractical and ineffective. Bullets alone may provide insufficient magnesium.

(6) *Better absorption.* Provision of long fibre by feeding hay, silage and straw has been considered to be effective in milk fever prevention. It slows passage of ingesta and may allow better absorption of magnesium where cows are on autumn grass.

(7) *Ionic balance.* Alteration of the ionic balance by increasing the acidity of the diet may facilitate absorption of calcium. The addition of magnesium sulphate or calcium chloride to hay or mineralized acid to silage are methods which have been used to produce "acid" diets. Such procedures have been successful in reducing the incidence of milk fever, but may

be of limited practical application. N.B. Increasing magnesium alone may not be sufficient to prevent milk fever if diet is too high in calcium, if cows are too fat, or if shelter is not provided in unfavourable weather.

VITAMIN D

Injection of large doses of vitamin D_3 has been used successfully to prevent milk fever. The response is rather slow and to be effective injections must be given between 8 and 3 days before calving. The difficulty of predicting accurate calving dates may restrict its use.

VITAMIN D ANALOGUES

I Hydroxy cholecalciferol is converted directly in the liver to the active 1,25 dihydroxy vitamin D_3 and bypasses the step II hydroxylation undergone by vitamin D in the kidney which is controlled by PTH. This analogue therefore acts more quickly than vitamin D_3 and this means that it can be used closer to calving (between 24 and 96 h before calving).

A combination of induction of calving and injection of vitamin D analogue has been used successfully when calving date is uncertain and cow is judged to be a "high risk" animal.

The use of vitamin D or its analogues may not be successful in prevention of milk fever if adequate magnesium is not available to the pregnant cow.

CALCIUM SOLUTION

Calcium solution is frequently given as a prophylactic measure to cows which are calving or are about to calve. Injudicious use of calcium at this time, e.g. large depots of calcium solution injected subcutaneously may be contraindicated because of the risk of suppression of the normal hormonal control mechanisms. Hypercalcaemia stimulates release of calcitonin, a hormone which depresses PTH production.

HOUSING

Housing of cows has been shown to reduce the incidence of milk fever in autumn-calving herds and should be considered if other preventative measures have proved to be ineffective.

In the longer term, it may be advisable to avoid rearing heifer replacements from cows which have had a history of severe milk fever. Unfortunately, it is the high-yielding cows which are more susceptible to milk fever!

FURTHER READING

Horst, R. F. (1986). *Journal Dairy Science* **69**, 606–616.
Sansom, B. F., Manston, R. & Vagg, M. J. (1983). *Veterinary Record* **112**, 447–449.

CHAPTER 13

The "Downer Cow"

TONY ANDREWS

INTRODUCTION

A most challenging problem for any cattle clinician is that of the recumbent cow. It requires expertise in deciding the correct prognosis and treatment. Cases can occur at any time, but most are associated with parturition. The aetiology is still not fully understood and cases of recumbency around parturition can involve metabolic disorders, toxaemia, injury during or following calving, and management.

Clinical examination in all cases needs to be thorough and involves many areas (Table 13.1). However, despite careful assessment and clinical inspection a positive diagnosis cannot be made in many animals and these are classified as "downer cows".

The downer cow has been defined in many ways. However, certain diagnostic signs, although arbitrary, need to be included as follows:

(1) The cow has been down longer than 24 h.
(2) The cow is not suffering from hypocalcaemia (in practical terms where blood samples have not been taken, this can be described as one having had two courses of treatment for the condition).

(3)   There is no diagnosible cause.
(4)   The animal is in sternal recumbency (Fig. 13.1).
(5)   It is usually related to the calving period.

AETIOLOGY

It is highly probable that there are many different causes which may result in a cow becoming recumbent. However, in many cases secondary damage is responsible for the downer cow problem, pressure damage resulting in obstruction of the blood supply causing ischaemic necrosis with muscle and

Table 13.1 Aids to diagnosis of the recumbent cow.

History

Was the calving difficult?
Had it got up since calving?
Did it have milk fever?
Had treatments been given by farmer?
How long had it been recumbent?
Had position changed since recumbent?
How long had it been in current position?
Is BSE in the herd?

Examination

Position of animal	Heart sounds intensity
Position of legs	Sensation fluid
Abnormal position of parts of the body	Any other abnormality
	Rectal
Degree of consciousness	Vaginal
Presence/absence of faeces	Rothera's test
Type of faeces	Response to calcium therapy
Respiratory rate, depth, type	Haematological examination (especially PCV)
Temperature	Biochemical blood examination –
Pulse-rate, character	CPK AST (SGOT) urea,
Vaginal discharge	creatinine, protein, magnesium,
Ruminations	calcium, phosphorus, glucose,
Tone of tail	potassium, sodium, ketones
Mucous membranes – colour, moistness	
Pupillary size and reflex	

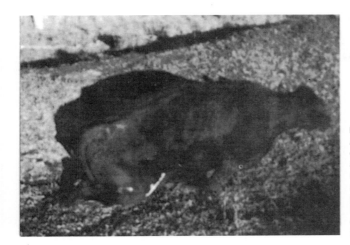

Fig. 13.1
A case of a downer cow in the crawler attitude. The animal recovered after administration of phosphorus. Photograph courtesy of Professor R. Penny.

nerve damage. This secondary damage can result in permanent recumbency even when the primary cause, commonly milk fever, has been successfully treated.

PATHOGENESIS

Many different factors may make the cow recumbent although most cases follow parturient paresis (Table 13.2). There is then compression of the soft tissues and when this continues it leads to nerve and muscle damage. Those muscles which are still functioning allow the animal to struggle causing muscle tearing and haemorrhage. The compression leads to obstruction of the blood supply in the distal part of the hindlimbs which in turn tends to lead to venous congestion stasis and thrombosis and then ischaemic necrosis with eventual permanent recumbency.

SIGNS

The typical downer cow is bright and alert. It will eat relatively well, drink normally, with normal urination and defecation.

Table 13.2 Some causes predisposing to "downer cow" syndrome.

Metabolic disorders	Toxaemia	Injuries during parturition	Injuries following parturition	Management
Hypocalcaemia	Peracute or acute mastitis	Ruptured uterus	Fractured pelvis	Malnutrition
Hypomagnesaemia		Internal haemorrhage	Fractured femur	Overfat
				Slippery floors in calving boxes
Hypophosphataemia	Metritis – acute septic	Obturator paralysis usually + poor flooring	Rupture of the round ligament	Delayed calcium therapy
Hypokalaemia	Acute diffuse peritonitis	Fractured pelvis	Dislocation of hip	Veterinary treatment (e.g. epidural anaesthesia)
		Sacral displacement	Rupture of adductor muscles	
Acetonaemia	Rupture of reticulum abomasum, uterus	Sciatic nerve paralysis		
Fat cow syndrome	Aspiration pneumonia	Exhaustion	Rupture of gastrocnemius muscle/tendon	*Others* Displaces abomasum (left or right) BSE Shock
Acidosis	Traumatic reticulitis/pericarditis		Damage to peripheral nerves, e.g. tibial	
Bloat			Pressure syndrome following milk fever	
Hypothermia (usually abroad)				

The rectal temperature is usually normal, as is the respiratory rate, but often the pulse rate is raised. Biochemical tests may show raised blood creatine phosphokinase and aspartate aminotransferase levels. If there is much muscle damage then there is proteinuria. If the cows are made to rise, the front legs can bear weight but the back legs are generally weaker.

PATHOLOGY

In most cases the upper adductor muscles of the hindlimb show haemolysis and degeneration. The muscles on the anterior border of the pelvis often present local ischaemic necrosis (Fig. 13.2). There is often associated oedema and haemorrhage around the major nerves (peroneal, obturator and sciatic). Commonly haemorrhages occur around the hip joint and in some cases the round ligament ruptures. The liver is often pale and fatty with the heart flabby.

PROGNOSIS

The most important decision any veterinary surgeon has to make on encountering a downer cow is what prognosis should be given. There is no complete answer to this problem, but a decision can be arrived at by considering: (a) known statistics of such cases; (b) the signs which are present; (c) the continual reassessment of the animal; (d) changes in biochemical enzyme levels; and (e) the attitude of the stockman.

STATISTICS

About half of all downer cows get up within 4 days of becoming recumbent. Once the animal has been down longer than 10 days the prognosis is poor. However, there are cases of individual animals returning to their feet after 2–3 weeks, or even a month!

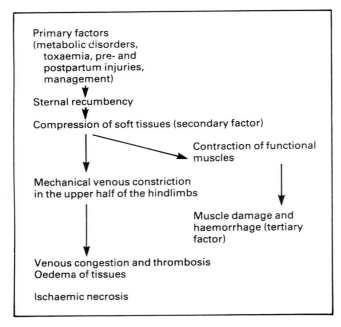

Fig. 13.2
Pathogenesis of ischaemic necrosis.

PRESENTING SIGNS

Each animal should be thoroughly assessed at the initial examination and any subsequent examination. Some of the signs and attitudes described in Tables 13.3 and 13.4 will give an indication of possible cause and prognosis. This may also help decide the possible laboratory investigations.

CONTINUAL REASSESSMENT

Any case involving the downer cow should be frequently reassessed. The interval between visits depends on economics but, in the early stages, it is best to visit the animal daily and then every 2–4 days. At each visit a full clinical examination should be performed and any changes noted. Such alterations will usually give an indication as to whether or not the animal is improving or deteriorating. Biochemical examination of the blood often shows the animals to be suffering from various metabolic disorders with few, if any, related clinical signs such

Table 13.3 Presenting position of the downer cow, its probable causes and prognosis.

Position or stance of animal	Cause	Prognosis
"Creeper" or "crawler" (attempts are made to rise with the hindquarters being lifted from the ground)	Hypocalcaemia, hypomagnesaemia, hypophosphataemia. Peroneal paralysis	Good
"Frog legged cow". The hindlimbs are partially flexed and displaced distally	Hypocalcaemia. Obturator paralysis. Tibial nerve damage. Adductor muscle damage	Mainly good
Hindlimbs rigidly extended rostrally so they are in contact with the elbows of the front legs. If the legs are placed in a normal position often they return to the stance	Often upper limb problems, e.g. hip dislocation, hip joint trauma, rupture of ligamentum teres. Muscular degeneration. Sciatic nerve damage	Hopeless
Rest on one side. If moved on to other side then returns to original position	May be damage to upper side but if due to muscle flaccidity then upper side is normal. Sciatic nerve damage. Peroneal paralysis. Pressure syndrome	Poor – depends very much on nursing
Legs extended behind the animal	Pubic damage. Nerve damage. Muscle damage	Usually poor

Table 13.4 Attitude changes in recumbent cattle.

Attitude	Positive cases	Prognosis
Lateral recumbency with head back	Chronic metabolic problems. Brain conditions or damage	Hopeless
Hyperaesthesia. Some show tetany or lateral recumbency	Mainly brain conditions or damage. Some have hypomagnesaemia or hypocalcaemia	Poor Good
Non-alert	Brain damage. Hypermagnesaemia (after therapy)	Poor

as hypocalcaemia, hypomagnesaemia, hypophosphataemia, secondary hypokalaemia and ketosis. In cases which appear to remain static the serum or plasma enzyme levels may be helpful.

BIOCHEMICAL ASSESSMENT

In all cases biochemical parameters should only be used as an assessment where clinical examination fails to indicate the cow's progress. Such interpretation should thus only be used in cows which appear to be the same at each visit. Various evaluations of results can be made but most based on single samples have proved unsuccessful. It would seem that there are no significant combinations which will provide a successful prognostic agent at the first examination, although a prognosis can be partly based on certain plasma enzyme levels rising or falling.

Testing and interpretation are based on taking samples starting after the animal has been down for longer than a day. The interval between successive tests should be greater than 24 h.

Unfortunately at present there is no prognostic agent which will give a reliable answer for about 2 days. Analysis of data derived from blood samples taken by British Cattle Veterinary Association members has shown that there is usually a fall in creatine phosphokinase after 2 days and in aspartate aminotransferase and urea after 3 days in recovered cattle, without a corresponding drop in those that have to be slaughtered. This study, which was conducted at Bristol University, suggested that a combination of condition score, quality of nursing and assessment of the levels of aspartate aminotransferase, creatine phosphokinase, magnesium and calcium accurately predicted the outcome of 86 % of cases 2 days after going down. The use of combined blood magnesium, urea and creatine phosphokinase levels, quality of nursing and whether the animal was attempting to rise correctly forecast the outcome in 92 % of cases sampled at 3 days.

STOCKMANSHIP

Finally, however excellent the veterinary surgeon's own powers of detection, treatment and prognosis, all will be to no avail if there is not adequate nursing. Bedding must also be sufficient. More animals outside tend to rise than those indoors and cows in good condition also have a better prognosis. Thus prognosis is as much dependent on the stockman as the cow.

TREATMENT

The good veterinary surgeon and stockman will be assessing the cow continually. Ideally the animal will need to be kept outside, preferably in a small flat paddock without a stream and near to the buildings. It can be hauled there on a gate or palette using a buck rake or with a cattle net and fore-end loader. If indoors, it should be bedded on deep manure or straw to give the animal purchase if it should attempt to rise. Where conditions are cramped the cow should be moved. If there is a tendency for the legs to straddle they can be kept together with a soft rope in a figure of eight, or hobbles (Somerset: Chard) (Save a Cow; Arnolds), or the use of two dog collars and rope. The cow should be fed and watered at least twice daily.

If in a field with other cattle the cow can be placed inside a ring feeder. If the weather is poor some form of shelter should be erected. The cow should be milked twice daily and turned from side to side an odd number of times to try and reduce the possibility of ischaemic muscle damage, hypostatic congestion and pneumonia. The problem with large modern herds is for the stockman to devote enough time to the cow without neglecting his obligations to the rest of the herd. These responsibilities in some cases are irreconcilable and in such cases slaughter may then be the only humane course.

Treatment must involve rectifying any metabolic deficiencies. The only therapeutic agent with a specific indication for use in the downer cow is tripelennamine hydrochloride (Vetibenzamine; Ciba Geigy). Some people use a Bagshawe hoist to move the animal, but this can cause damage, particularly with pelvic injuries. Another method is a supportive harness (Downacow Harness; Alfred Murray). Over recent years several inflatable bags have become available (Bovijac; Alfred Cox), (Henshaw Air Lift; J. M. Henshaw) (Downer Cow Cushion; Hamco Products). These have the advantage of being relatively comfortable and support the cow's body and allow limb circulation to be restored but with some the cow will fall off. The cow should remain raised for about half an hour. If a Bagshawe hoist is used it might best be undertaken in conjunction with an inflatable bag. The main advice to give is that all cases of recumbent cows should be treated correctly, sufficiently and promptly.

CHAPTER 14

Summer Mastitis – the Current Position

J. ERIC HILLERTON

INTRODUCTION

Summer mastitis affects 20–60 % of dairy farms in England and Wales. It usually affects the same herds from year to year, so that 40 % rarely experience the problem. Even more farms in northern Europe suffer and from a much higher incidence. What is the problem, what does it cost and how can it be prevented?

CLINICAL DISEASE

The disease is fairly easily recognized (Table 14.1) but, frequently, diagnosis is too late to allow treatment sufficiently effective to retain secretory function of the affected quarter(s). The most comon sequel is a "blind quarter".

Given early diagnosis and rapid and sustained treatment the prognosis for recovery of the affected animal is good. Occasionally some secretory function may be retained. If treatment is delayed or withheld the animal becomes seriously ill. In addition to an extreme mastitis pyrexia, lethargy and inappetence will develop. Lameness and joint swelling,

Table 14.1 Diagnosis of summer mastitis.

Early stages in dry animals
  Lethargy, loss of appetite, no cudding and a solitary animal at pasture
  Inflamed and swollen teat, close inspection shows that the gland is
    affected too
  Animal particularly attractive to flies

Early stages in newly calved cattle
  Obviously abnormal secretion, foul smelling, thick and creamy or with
    many clots; quarter hot and swollen

Later stages
  Quarter hot, swollen and brick hard
  Secretion purulent and foul smelling
  Elevated temperature
  Lameness progressing from hind legs
  Swelling of joints
  Possible abortion
  Toxaemia

---

particularly of the hind limbs, often follows and rupture of
mammary abscesses is common. The bacteraemia/toxaemia
may be fatal (1–2 %) and some animals will abort. Perinatal
death is substantially increased and calves born live frequently
do not thrive.

Successful management of summer mastitis requires early
identification by the stockman which can only come from
close scrutiny of animals at risk. This is uncommon. The non-
lactating stock are usually pastured remotely from the main
farm site and outbreaks of the disease tend to occur when
there is maximum pressure on the staff from harvesting. There
can be no substitute for close and frequent observation of
stock.

It is unlikely that diagnosis by bacteriology will ever be of
much value as treatment must start immediately. Recent
evidence showed that 80 % of diagnoses of summer mastitis
by farmers were correct. The other cases were caused by other
bacteria (e.g. *Streptococcus uberis*) more likely to respond to
antibiotic treatment. Probably the foul odour of organic acids
and indole in the secretion, produced by *Peptococcus indolicus*,
is the most reliable diagnostic feature. Only where drastic
action such as teat amputation or immediate culling occurs
are there important economic consequences of misdiagnosis.

TREATMENT

A number of different approaches to treatment have been tried, from immediate culling, or teat amputation, to intramammary infusion with proteolytic enzymes or frequent application of antibiotics. Successful bacteriological cure of summer mastitis is rare in the dry period.

There is no panacea and, in trials in different European countries, secretory function rarely returned. Therapy is most important in keeping the animal clinically healthy. The best therapy is to treat the animal with antibiotics intramuscularly, strip the quarter frequently and apply intramammary antibiotics in the evening. The therapy must be continued for at least 5 days and the infected animal must be quarantined immediately. It is a source of further infection.

EPIDEMIOLOGY

The incidence of summer mastitis varies markedly within the UK. Generally the problem is greater in more intensive dairying areas. This may be because there is a higher density of animals at risk or because of some relationship with better grassland. The Dutch, Germans and Danes suggest that summer mastitis is associated with sandy soils and many British farmers find most cases on "green sand". The high humus content, open structure and free-draining of these soils are particularly suitable for foraging, soil-dwelling, insect larvae.

Summer mastitis is considered to be epidemiologically most severe in northern maritime Europe. It is also prevalant in Japan and Florida where an incidence of 5 % has been reported. It has also been reported less frequently in several other parts of the USA, Greece, Australia, Zimbabwe and Brazil.

The epidemiology may vary in all of these dairy industries but there are a number of common features:

(1) Infection is most common in late gestation and at calving.
(2) Specialized dairy breeds are more susceptible.

(3)   Older cows are more susceptible (Fig. 14.1).
(4)   There is an annual variation in incidence – a 3-year cycle has been reported from the Netherlands and the UK.
(5)   Some countries have a distinct seasonal pattern.

The seasonal pattern (Fig. 14.2) is probably related to calving pattern and to fly incidence as described later. In Eire, where spring calving predominates, one third of cases occur in the spring. There is also a significant spring peak of incidence in England and Wales independent of calving rate. This may be another example of the influence of density of animals at risk.

AETIOLOGY

Bacteriological analysis of summer mastitis secretion shows a complex infection. Usually *Corynebacterium pyogenes* predominates and the severity of infection is related to the presence of anaerobes (Fig. 14.3). *Peptococcus indolicus* is the most common anaerobe, but *Bacteroides melanogenicus* and *Fusobacterium necrophorum* are often found.

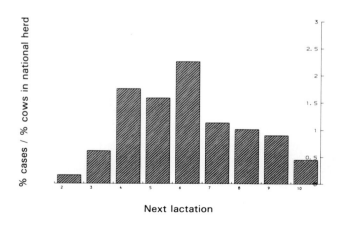

Fig. 14.1 Susceptibility to summer mastitis with age at next lactation of dry cows.

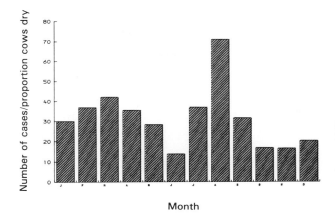

Fig. 14.2
Summer mastitis
incidence from VIDA
returns 1975–1986
weighted by
proportion of national
herd dry in any
month.

Much of the reported variation (Table 14.2) in anaerobe isolation is caused by different diagnostic criteria – Sweden and Holland include all uncalved-heifer mastitis in their definition. Crucially there are differences in the methodology employed for bacterial sampling and culturing.

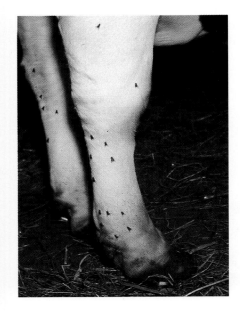

Fig. 14.3
Dry cow infected with *C. pyogenes* and *P. indolicus* showing swollen hind legs.

Table 14.2 Recoveries of bacteria (% cases).

Species	UK	Denmark	FDR	Australia	Sweden	Holland
Corynebacterium pyogenes	85	72	89	81	40	37
Peptococcus indolicus	62	87	69	48	39	33
Streptococcus dysgalactiae	24	37	40	16	39	8
Stuart–Schwann cocci	22	83	–	52	24	–
Bacteroides melanogenicus	<1	35	–	23	–	8
Fusobacterium necrophorum	1	51	–	74	–	22

PATHOGENESIS

The severity of infection varies with the bacteria involved, but extensive damage to the secretory tissue occurs (Fig. 14.4).

Experimental work from Denmark has shown that *P. indolicus* enhances the production and activity of *C. pyogenes* haemolysin. There are a number of virulence factors (haemolysin, coagulase, hyaluronidase) produced by the bacteria involved in summer mastitis and synergism is to be expected.

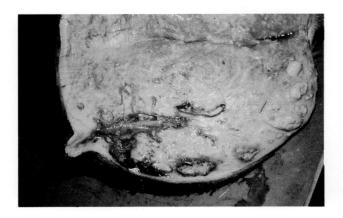

Fig. 14.4
Section of mastitic udder.

The route of invasion of the udder by a mixture of bacteria is unknown but it seems unlikely that simultaneous invasion by up to five species of bacteria occurs. Experimentally, infections can be induced by inoculation via the teat duct or exposure of the teat surface to a large number of bacteria. Evidence for the teat route being important in natural infections comes from the frequency of summer mastitis following teat damage. Work at Compton has shown, using the teat duct route, that *C. pyogenes* can be imposed on *P. indolicus* infections and vice versa with a consequent increase in clinical severity.

However opinions differ on the mechanism of invasion. There are a number of possibilities:

(1) Bacteria contaminating the teat skin or orifice invade through the teat duct.
(2) Invasion following the development of an infected skin lesion.
(3) Bacteria enter the gland by draining via the supramammary lymph node from other infected lesions.
(4) Bacteria invaded by haematogenous spread from other sites.

It must be remembered that *C. pyogenes* and *P. indolicus* are ubiquitous in the bovine, easily recoverable from mucous membranes and particularly from abscesses in cattle. Quite possibly a number of routes occur in practice.

Clinical mastitis, virtually identical to summer mastitis, can occur in the lactating gland, but many cases reported in lactation originate in the dry period only to be discovered after calving. Experimental work has shown that infection by *C. pyogenes, P. indolicus* and both together are more easily established and are more severe in the dry gland (Fig. 14.5).

VECTOR TRANSMISSION

It is a long and widely held belief that flies transmit summer mastitis. There is considerable circumstantial evidence to support this:

(1) The peak incidence of disease occurs when flies are most frequent on cattle (Fig. 14.6).

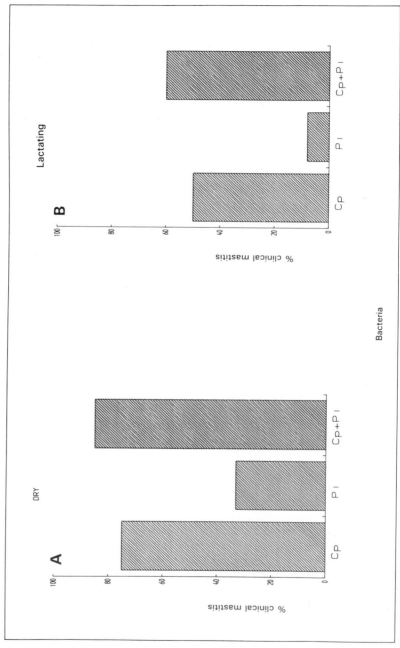

Fig. 14.5 Experimental infections with *C. pyogenes* (Cp) and, or *P. indolicus* (Pi) in dry cows (A) or lactating cows (B).

(2)   The sheep headfly, *Hydrotaea irritans* (Figs 14.7 and 14.8), is the most frequent visitor to the teats of cattle and flies carry mixtures of summer mastitis-causing bacteria (Fig. 14.9).
(3)   The characteristic epidemiological spread of disease coincides with the geographical distribution of the fly.
(4)   Control of flies reduces the incidence of summer mastitis.
(5)   Infections are commoner in front quarters which flies can reach more easily.

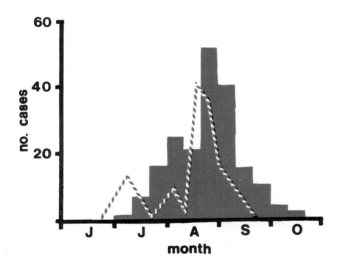

Fig. 14.6
Pattern of occurrence of summer mastitis in a 1984 survey, July, August and September, (histogram) correlates with the numbers of *Hydrotaea irritans* visiting the teats of pregnant heifers (line).

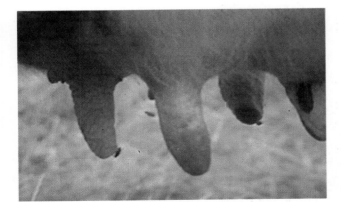

Fig. 14.7
Hydrotora irritans on and around heifer teats.

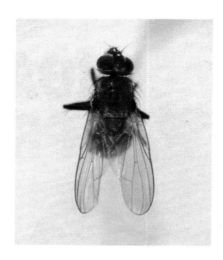

Fig. 14.8
Hydrotaea irritans.

On the contrary:

(1) "Summer mastitis" is frequent outside the fly season.
(2) The disease occurs in regions where neither *Hydrotaea irritans* nor a readily identifiable substitute occurs.
(3) Numerous attempts in Britain, Denmark, The Netherlands

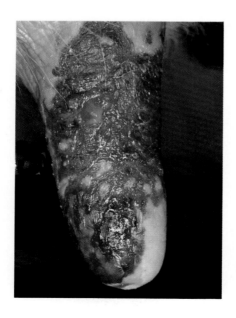

Fig. 14.9
Teat "summer sore" – the consequence of a
teat lesion followed by licking and fly attack.

and West Germany to transmit the disease using flies have failed despite earlier unsubstantiated reports of success.

It is likely that *H. irritans* is involved in secondary transmission in the summer peak of disease but that other mechanisms operate. Thus isolated cases will occur at any time of the year following invasion of the gland from an infected teat lesion, gross contamination of the teat or endogenous spread from another focus. Further cases in the herd may arise from this source of either (a) mechanical transfer via bedding, bodily contact, etc., or (b) mechanical transfer of bacteria by flies from infected animals to others. It has been shown that flies can retain the bacteria in the gut for several days and represent them during subsequent feeding bouts.

The occurrence of the epidemiological explosion of cases will be governed by:

(1) The rate of transfer – much increased by flies.
(2) The number and density of animals at risk – cases are more frequent when there are more animals at risk.
(3) The susceptibility of animals – stage of gestation.
(4) Perhaps the stress on the cattle. Factors involved might include the level/quality of nutrition, late gestation/calving and fly pestation all working to compromise the immune defences.

CONTROL

There are well-recognized means of reducing the incidence of summer mastitis:

(1) Use dry cow treatment on all cows and repeat after 3 weeks where there is a history of summer mastitis.
(2) Control flies from July to September by persistent methods – ear-tags or pour-ons.
(3) Treat all teat lesions and trauma promptly to limit fly attack.
(4) Consider teat bandages or repellents applied to teats.
(5) Avoid high risk pastures.
(6) Feed animals properly.

(7)   Perhaps change the calving pattern.
(8)   Monitor animals, a close inspection at least twice daily, and segregate any suspect animals *immediately*.

Good results have been obtained with long acting antibiotics for almost 40 years. They remain indispensable, reducing infection rates by up to 80 %. Frequently one application is insufficient and should be repeated after 3–4 weeks, but well before the expected calving date.

The teat should be protected from damage and bacterial contamination. Flies are well controlled by the synthetic pyrethroid insecticides but two medicated ear-tags per animal are needed to control flies on the teats. Ear-tags and pour-on formulations are more labour efficient, longer acting and probably, safer too. Belgian work has shown that ear-tags reduced incidence in heifers by 75 %. They are to be preferred to trying to infuse heifers with antibiotics, especially by the unskilled.

Barriers (e.g. Stockholm tar) are another long-established method for control of summer mastitis. However, controlled efficacy data are not available. Teat bandages have been used effectively in Denmark, emphasizing the likely role of the fly and teat damage in the pathogenesis of the disease.

There have been over 20 attempts, over 75 years, to vaccinate against summer mastitis, none producing convincing evidence of protection from infection, although there is evidence of a reduction in severity. German workers have successfully vaccinated mice but failed to protect calves. Work at Compton and elsewhere has shown that *C. pyogenes* invoke a poor and short-lived immune response, even after clinical mastitis.

ECONOMICS

The costs of summer mastitis for England and Wales, Denmark and Belgium have been determined (Table 14.3).

Of practical importance is the cost benefit of control measures. It is difficult to construct a complete assessment taking into account all types of control and the proportion of cost which should be accredited to the measure, e.g. fly control might reduce summer mastitis but it will also control other

Table 14.3 Estimated costs of summer mastitis.

Type of animal	Denmark in-calf	England & Wales dry cow	Belgium average milker
Cost per animal (£)	444	450	296
National incidence (%)	5.0	1.5	2.0
Cost per group (£M)	2.4	10.0	0.5
National cost for all groups (£M) (1988 values)	11.5	15.0	0.9

fly problems and influence productivity.

A simple analysis is given here for the effect on the incidence of summer mastitis in dry cows using published UK figures and 1988 costs (Table 14.4). A similar calculation could be made for the other effective control measures showing benefits. However they will not be additive and the best strategy, an integrated programme of some sort, would need to be calculated for each set of circumstances.

FUTURE

There are a number of additional areas concerning summer mastitis where little is known and much remains to be

Table 14.4 Cost benefit for dry cow antibiotic prevention of summer mastitis using repeated infusion of antibiotic.

Treatment	Incidence (%)	Cost for a herd of 100 cows at risk (£)		
		Loss	Cost of DCT	Total cost
None	9.8	4410	0	4410
Repeat DCT	3.0	1350	480	1830

Cost: Benefit of a repeat infusion in a high-risk area = 2.4:1 or a saving of over £25 per cow investigated. Perhaps it will be possible soon to have more information on the effects of:

(1)   Nutrition and stress affecting susceptibility to infection. Incidence is highest when stress is high and nutrition less than best.
(2)   Resistance to insecticides. This has been reported from USA and Belgium and is suspected in Germany. New products and integrated control strategies may be needed soon.
(3)   Teat barriers. These remain to be tested and more refined methods may be possible.
(4)   Calving pattern. Economic forces may reduce the benefits of autumn calving. Reduced incidence following early summer calving may tip the economic argument.
(5)   Vaccines. A long-term aim must remain to produce a vaccine. A vaccine against the virulence factors seems more likely than an anti-C. *pyogenes* product.

FURTHER READING

Thomas, G., Over, H. J., Vecht, U. & Nansen, P. (eds) (1987). *Summer Mastitis*. The proceedings of an EEC workshop on summer mastitis. Nijhoff, Dordrecht.

CHAPTER 15

Differential Diagnosis of Chronic Ruminal Tympany in Cattle

JIM PINSENT

INTRODUCTION

The differential diagnosis of chronic and subacute ruminal tympany in cattle is not always straightforward. It is helpful to remember that all conditions producing these signs must fall into one or other of two main groups: first those which interfere with normal ruminoreticular tone and motility and, secondly, those causing partial obstruction to the escape of gas from the rumen, motility and tone remaining normal.

CONDITIONS WHICH INTERFERE WITH NORMAL RUMINORETICULAR TONE AND MOTILITY

CHRONIC INFLAMMATORY LESIONS OF THE WALL OF RETICULUM AND OESOPHAGEAL GROOVE

Actinobacillosis of the reticulum and/or oesophageal groove

This most important disease produces a smooth raised painless and fibrous area or plaque, devoid of mucous membrane in the wall of the reticulum or the groove. The effect is to interfere with both eructation and rumination. There is usually a low-grade ruminal tympany which tends to be more pronounced after feeding, but is never completely absent, and although appetite is relatively normal, a slow weight loss occurs. Eructation is abnormal and incomplete and, if the oesophageal groove is badly affected, there may be a prolonged retching and gurgling noise associated with laboured attempts to bring up the first bolus of a new period of rumination.

Lesions are easily found at exploratory laparotomy, although this should not be necessary, for this is one condition where treatment may be regarded almost as a diagnostic technique. Response to iodides, sulphonamides, and certain of the antibiotics (streptomycin/penicillin combinations or oxytetracyclines) is generally straightforward and successful if sufficiently prolonged. Sulphonamide or antibiotic therapy should be administered for at least 10 days, while iodide treatment should continue for 3–4 weeks.

Infected lacerations and partial penetrations of the mucous membrane of the reticulum and oesophageal groove

These may result from sharp foreign bodies, such as pieces of wire, tin, etc. These injuries lead to inflammatory thickening and *Corynebacterium pyogenes* abscessation – the foreign bodies themselves falling back into the reticulum. Such abscesses, partly buried in reactionary tissue, may frequently be opened and drained with a finger or the beak of an embryotomy knife at rumenotomy.

MUCH MORE IMPORTANT, HOWEVER, ARE CONDITIONS INVOLVING PERITONITIS

Any inflammatory change involving the peritoneal lining or rumen, reticulum, or even abomasum may lead to low grade motility or even atony of the rumen–reticulum.

Traumatic reticuloperitonitis

The classic syndrome in this group is, of course, traumatic reticuloperitonitis or "wire", now less commonly seen than in the immediate post-war years. Even in longstanding cases where some degree of rumen movement has returned, mild chronic ruminal tympany is frequently present, often superimposed on low-grade ruminal impaction, but with sufficient ruminorecticular movement to produce a positive reticular grunt test, usually spoken of as the Williams test.

Peptic abomasal ulceration

Peptic abomasal ulceration may well be without signs but once the ulcer has eroded sufficiently to involve the peritoneal lining, adhesions to omentum will form in the areas of the omentum. Abomasal tone and motility will be affected, with consequent adverse effects upon the tone and motility of the rumen and reticulum. It is not uncommon to find that such a cow undergoes perforation of the abomasal wall at the point of adhesion, but that the perforation is sealed by omental fat. The resulting syndrome includes intermittent low-grade pain, abnormal or negligible ruminoreticular movement, loss of weight, intermittent diarrhoea, and intermittent slight ruminal tympany which is only present at times when the cow is feeling sufficiently well to show a slightly improved appetite.
　　The other complications of peptic ulceration are unlikely to cause differential difficulty. A haemorrhagic abomasal ulcer

produces profound anaemia, but not tympany, while abomasal displacement with left flank adhesions may result in mild abomasal tympany, but is easily identified on auscultation or by the "push–splash" ballottement test.

Perforation of a peptic ulcer through abomasal wall in an area not covered by omentum may produce marked peritoneal tympany, but the syndrome is so acute and rapidly fatal that the question of differentiation from chronic ruminal tympany does not arise.

ACIDOSIS

Acidosis is due, primarily, to excess levels of fermentable energy feeds, producing a degree of ruminal acidosis which is highest after concentrate feeding. The classic acidotic condition is barley poisoning but, until the introduction of quotas, a degree of acidosis was constant in the ruminal environment of many high-yielding and highly fed cows in early lactation. The slight ruminal tympany and excessively soft faeces plus suboptimal appetite and milk yield were familiar features in early lactating cows, in which ruminal acidosis after each parlour feed resulted in a varying degree of ruminal atony.

The majority of herds today have a much reduced concentrate ration and herd acidosis has become relatively uncommon, although it still occurs in those herds receiving higher levels of concentrate feed.

VAGUS INDIGESTION

Vagus indigestion is, in its usual manifestation, an extreme form of atony involving rumen, reticulum, and abomasum. It is caused by interference with the vagal innervation of their medial walls by peritoneal adhesions following foreign body penetration of the medial wall of the reticulum. In most such cases, the rumen fills up with, and becomes distended by, fluid formed largely by saliva and drinking water, in which float collections of food material. In occasional cases, however, a great deal of gas collects producing a very marked, but chronic and lasting, ruminal tympany.

TETANUS

Tetanus involves tonic spasm of the reticuloruminal musculature leading to chronic ruminal tympany. Although this tympany may be a very noticeable feature, even to the extent that the client's complaint may be that he has a cow with chronic bloat, rather than anything else, a routine examination will quickly reveal the raised tail, stiff movement, erect ears, and some degree of trismus, which lead one's thoughts to tetanus. Dehydration is frequently very noticeable, while most cases are constipated.

CHILL

It is sometimes forgotten in these days of piped water and drinking bowls that there are still some herds in which cows, during the winter, are turned out to drink from water troughs in the yard twice daily, there being no drinking bowls in many old cowsheds. During the winter months this water may well be at, or about, freezing point and the chill effect when a large quantity is drunk quickly by thirsty cows may produce ruminal atony of several hours' duration. It was by no means unusual in such circumstances for veterinary assistance to be summoned to treat what appeared as a herd problem of chronic tympany.

A similar, but less-noticeable syndrome, may occur if cows take in large quantities of frosted grass in early spring, but as dairy herds are rarely turned out by night until late April or early May, this syndrome is relatively uncommon.

CONDITIONS WHICH CAUSE PARTIAL OBSTRUCTION TO THE ESCAPE OF GAS FROM THE RETICULUM AND RUMEN, MOTILITY AND TONE BEING LARGELY NORMAL

OESOPHAGEAL WALL LESIONS, USUALLY TRAUMATIC IN ORIGIN

Oesophageal stricture

Oesophageal stricture is usually the result of encircling lesions of the mucous membrane, and possibly muscular layers, caused by temporary obstruction by a roughly spheroidal body such as a potato, or a portion of fodder beet. Equally, the damage may result from rough and amateurish attempts to remove such an object from a low cervical or intrathoracic site.

Oesophageal wall abscesses

Oesophageal wall abscesses are usually traumatic in origin.

Oesophageal dilatation

Oesophageal dilatation usually results from trauma affecting the mucous and muscular layers. A pouch forms, usually in a low cervical position just anterior to the thoracic inlet. This fills up with food, which then obstructs the oesophagus, which may fill with food above this point producing long-lasting moderate ruminal tympany. The dilatation in the oesophagus may, when full, be visible from the exterior.

Papillomata

Papillomata at the cardia are not uncommon and may interfere with the escape of ruminal gas.

Paralysis of central origin

Listerellosis (listeriosis) among other nervous signs, including incoordination, aggressive behaviour, circling and pyrexia, usually produces paralysis of the facial cranial nerve (seventh). Occasionally, however, other cranial nerves are affected and among the clinical signs may be pharyngeal paralysis with collection of food material in the back of the mouth and the pharynx. This may be sufficiently severe to cause a partly open mouth, drooling saliva, choking "gagging" sounds, and a degree of ruminal tympany which admittedly is practically insignificant considering the severe nature of the nervous signs.

LESIONS CAUSING EXTERNAL PRESSURE ON THE OESOPHAGUS WILL PRODUCE CHRONIC TYMPANY

Thymic lymphosarcoma

Thymic lymphosarcoma occasionally causes mediastinal space-occupying lesions in young cattle, along with bilaterally symmetrical enlargement of lymph nodes, a raised pulse rate, muffled heart sounds and some degree of dyspnoea. The neoplastic mass is sometimes palpable at the thoracic inlet, causes significant ruminal tympany, and is visible on radiographs should the procedure be considered viable from the economic angle, or practical in the farm environment.

Enlargement of lymph nodes

Enlargement of the posterior mediastinal lymph nodes is an important cause of chronic tympany and is usually caused by one of three organisms:

(1)   *Corynebacterium pyogenes*
(2)   Actinobacillus
(3)   Tuberculosis

In cases in which there is no obvious reason for chronic

ruminal tympany, it is worthwhile embarking upon a course of treatment with an antibiotic such as penicillin–streptomycin mixture. Actinobacillosis will probably respond; *C. pyogenes* may show some degree of response, while tuberculosis is hopefully very unlikely today.

Diaphragmatic hernia

Diaphragmatic hernia in cattle produces a variable clinical picture. The most common syndrome appears to result from traumatic reticulitis, the reticulum passing, at least in part, through a hernial opening which develops in post-reticulitis diaphragmatic adhesions. The clinical picture is of low-grade anterior abdominal/posterior thoracic pain more or less similar to that of reticulitis itself. There will also be, of course, interference with eructation and possibly with reticulo-ruminal motility itself, leading to chronic ruminal tympany. Later vagus indigestion may develop as a result of vagal nerve involvement as it passes through the diaphragm.

Botulism

In recent years an increasing number of cases believed to be caused by botulism have been reported in various parts of the country. Unless one works in the vicinity of specialized laboratory facilities and expertise, it is very difficult to substantiate such a diagnosis. The clinical picture would appear to include lassitude and general muscle weakness, recumbency, constipation, lack of tone in the tail, difficult prehension and mastication, and difficulty in ruminating and eructating which become cumbersome and noisy procedures and then cease altogether. A low-grade ruminal tympany develops superimposed upon a scanty hard rumen content. This condition falls into both the main aetiological groups.

DIAGNOSIS OF CHRONIC AND SUBACUTE RUMINAL TYMPANY

The diagnosis of chronic and subacute ruminal tympany in cattle depends first upon a careful routine clinical examination to assess the more general signs, if any, which may accompany the tympany. First one must decide whether the tympany is related to a specific alimentary condition, or whether it is associated with lack of gastric tone due to a more general disease.

If satisfied that the condition is primarily alimentary, then one must differentiate between lack of ruminoreticular movement and oesophageal obstruction. At this point, one must be sure that the tympany is ruminal in origin – it is not particularly unusual to find sufficient gas in an abomasum displaced to the left to produce an impression of left flank tympany. Careful auscultation should leave one in no doubt, although it is not always easy to distinguish between the sounds of left displacement of a gas-filled abomasum, early vagus indigestion, and actinobacillosis of the reticular wall.

Once satisfied that the tympany is ruminal, then theoretically the passage of an endoscope down the oesophagus under careful restraint and good sedation, using the equine approach via the nasal chamber, should be very helpful. Unfortunately, even clinicians who possess such an endoscope and are conversant with its use are unlikely to risk a very expensive piece of equipment in the examination of a cow probably worth less than the endoscope in the prevailing conditions of modern cattle practice. If this is the case, then passage of a probang with great care, or a stomach tube (much safer, but less informative) is the next best thing, although the information obtained is only too often inconclusive.

A surgical rumen fistula in the left sublumbar fossa may be helpful to release gas and thus aid ruminal tone, or to allow ease of rehydration should this be necessary, but is no help in diagnosis.

Exploratory left flank laparotomy is the most satisfactory of the available diagnostic techniques in difficult cases, for it is a safe and simple technique which allows manual exploration of a very large part of the abdomen, and then via a rumenotomy incision, of the rumen, reticulum, oesophageal groove, reticulo-omasal orifice, cardia, and the lower 7–10 cm of the oesophagus at which point simultaneous passage of a stomach tube is often very helpful.

It is unfortunate that prevalent attitudes today tend to ignore laparotomy and rumenotomy as diagnostic aids, maintaining that it is unjustified to use such techniques until diagnosis and prognosis have been made, and success guaranteed. The assumption often seems to be that the butcher is a better economic proposition than the surgeon!

Unfortunately, laboratory assistance plays little part in the differential diagnosis of chronic tympany, apart from the general rule that a white cell picture with less than 10 000 cells/mm^3 total count, and less than 50 % total neutrophils, is unlikely if lesions of peritonitis are present.

FURTHER READING

Williams, E. I. (1955) *Veterinary Record* **907**, 922.

CHAPTER 16

Differential Diagnosis of Diarrhoea in Adult Cattle

LYALL PETRIE

INTRODUCTION

The importance of diarrhoea as a clinical sign in adult cows can be illustrated from a survey of more than 400 adult cattle (i.e. cattle over 2 years old) admitted to the University of Glasgow Veterinary School over a 2-year period. Of 404 adult cattle, 31 % were diarrhoeic on admission and diarrhoea was the major presenting sign in 20 %.

The diseases in which diarrhoea occurs as a major clinical finding, those conditions in which oral lesions are found and the major differential features of the diseases are presented in Tables 16.1–16.4.

Diarrhoea also occurs in diseases such as chronic congestive cardiac failure, lead poisoning, left abomasal displacement and acute coliform mastitis in which it is not a major presenting sign. These conditions will not be discussed in this article. Passing reference only will be made to several plant poisonings which are not common.

Table 16.1 Major causes of diarrhoea in adult cattle.

Acute conditions	*Chronic conditions*
Salmonellosis	Johne's disease
Winter dysentery	Mucosal disease
Overeating acidosis	Ostertagiasis
Malignant catarrhal fever	Renal amyloidosis
Ragwort poisoning	Upper alimentary tract squamous cell carcinoma
Arsenic poisoning	Alimentary lymphosarcoma/other alimentary tumour
Mucosal disease	Abdominal fat necrosis
	Molybdenosis

Table 16.2 Diarrhoea in adult cattle: conditions with oral lesions.

Mucosal disease
Malignant catarrhal fever
Upper alimentary tract squamous cell carcinoma

ACUTE CONDITIONS

SALMONELLOSIS

With the introduction of the Zoonosis Order in 1975, the incidence of salmonellosis in Britain is well tabulated. During the past 10 years there have been 400–800 salmonella incidents annually in adult cattle. The majority of incidents are caused by either *Salmonella typhimurium* or *S. dublin*. Although *S. typhimurium* predominates, any *Salmonella* species serotype can give rise to serious outbreaks of salmonellosis.

The clinical syndrome produced following infection with any of the *Salmonella* species serotypes is very similar. However, there are major differences in the epizootiology of the two most prevalent serotypes, *S. dublin* and *S. typhimurium*. *S. typhimurium* is an ubiquitous organism which can infect many species, whereas *S. dublin* is almost host specific for cattle.

Table 16.3 Differential diagnosis of diarrhoea in adult cattle: acute conditions.

Condition	Presenting signs	Epidemiology	Other significant clinical and laboratory findings	Diagnosis
Salmonellosis	Dysentery. Depression. Decreased milk yield, Anorexia	Group problem. Both dairy and beef, mainly dairy cattle. All ages affected	Pyrexia (40–41°C). Tachypnoea. Tachycardia. Rumen stasis. Faeces may contain shreds of epithelium, fibrinous casts. Abortion. Mortality can be high	Clinical signs. Faecal culture. Post-mortem findings.
Winter dysentery	Very sudden onset. Profuse, watery black diarrhoea. Marked drop in milk yield	Group problem. Milking dairy cows, often 100% of herd. Early winter, 2–3 weeks after housing	No pyrexia. Decreased appetite. No mortality. Diarrhoea may contain small spots of blood. Short duration	Clinical signs. Rapid recovery in 2–3 days without treatment
Overeating acidosis	Depression. Ataxia. Faeces soft to profuse diarrhoea. Abdominal distension	One to several animals affected. History of access to grain or concentrates	Rumen stasis. Dilated pupils, slow pupillary response. Tachycardia. Dehydration. Subnormal temperature. Malodorous faeces, may contain obvious grain. Rumen pH<5. No rumen protozoa	Clinical signs. History of access to grain/concentrates. Decreased rumen, pH<5

continued

Table 16.3 Continued

Condition	Presenting signs	Epidemiology	Other significant clinical and laboratory findings	Diagnosis
Malignant catarrhal fever	Oculonasal discharge. Severe depression. Anorexia. Scanty to profuse diarrhoea	Single animal. Both dairy and beef cattle. Often young adult. May have association with lambing sheep and therefore occur in spring and early summer	Hyperaemic, erosive mouth lesions. Pyrexia. Bilateral corneal opacity. Photophobia. Enlarged lymph nodes. Haematuria. Frequent micturition. Encephalitis	Clinical signs. Post-mortem findings
Ragwort poisoning	Black, tarry diarrhoeic faeces. Straining. Prolapse of rectum. Depression	Single to several animals depending on source. Both dairy and beef cattle. All ages affected	Decreased appetite. Normal temperature. Jaundice. Ascites* CNS signs – depression, ataxia. Weight loss. Liver function values variable. Mild hypoalbuminaemia. Hyperammonaemia	Clinical signs. Laboratory data. Liver biopsy. Post-mortem findings

Arsenic poisoning	Sudden death. Marked depression. Abdominal pain. Profuse diarrhoea which may contain blood and shreds of epithelium	Group problem. All breeds affected. Any age. Access to arsenic	Anorexia. Tachycardia. Normal temperature. Death within 12–36 h of onset. Arsenic detectable in urine	Clinical signs. History of access. Liver arsenic levels >10–15 ppm. Detectable arsenic in urine
Mucosal disease	Diarrhoea. Depression. Weight loss. Oculonasal discharge. Lameness	Single animal. Both dairy and beef cattle. Less than 4 years old	Hyperaemia of oral mucous membranes. Small irregular erosions on hard palate. Linear fissures at commissures of lips. Salivation. Interdigital ulceration. Skin lesions. Anorexia	Clinical signs. Virus isolation from blood, nasal swabs. Serology. Post-mortem findings

*Frequently possible to detect fluid thrill across abdomen owing to oedematous mesentery and intestines; only small volumes of free ascitic fluid.

Table 16.4 Differential diagnosis of diarrhoea in adult cattle: chronic conditions.

Condition	Presenting signs	Epidemiology	Other significant clinical and laboratory findings	Diagnosis
Johne's disease	Profuse diarrhoea. Weight loss. Bright. Good appetite	Single animal. Both dairy and beef cattle, 4–7 years old	Homogeneous faeces. Progressive weight loss. Good appetite until terminal. Non-pyrexic. Decreased milk yield. Clumps of acid-fast bacilli in 50 % of cases. Hypoalbuminaemia, <20 g/l. Anaemia – packed cell volume 25 % approximately	Clinical signs. Clumps of acid-fast bacilli in faecal smear. Post-mortem findings. Serology of limited value
Ostertagiasis	Profuse diarrhoea. Weight loss. Decreased milk yield	Group problem. Both dairy and beef cattle. Any age. Type 1 disease – autumn. Type 2 disease – spring/early summer	Appetite may be depressed. Normal temperature. Hypoalbuminaemia. Increased serum pepsinogen values >3000 miu. Faecal trichostrongyle egg counts high in Type 1 disease; low in Type 2 disease	Clinical signs. Serum pepsinogen values >3000 miu. Faecal egg counts. Epidemiology

Mucosal disease	Diarrhoea. Depression. Weight loss. Oculonasal discharge. Lameness	Single animal. Both dairy and beef cattle. Less than 4 years old	Hyperaemia of oral mucous membranes. Small irregular erosions on hard palate. Linear fissures at commissures of lips. Salivation. Interdigital ulceration. Skin lesions. Anorexia	Clinical signs. Virus isolation from blood, nasal swabs. Serology. Post-mortem findings
Renal amyloidosis	Profuse diarrhoea. Marked subcutaneous oedema. Good condition initially	Single animal. Middle aged dairy cows	Normal temperature. Decreased appetite. Decreased milk yield. Enlarged kidney. Proteinuria, 400–1200 mg/dl. Hypoalbuminaemia, <10 g/l. Increased plasma urea levels	Clinical signs. Proteinuria and hypoalbuminaemia. Post-mortem findings – massively enlarged kidneys

continued

Table 16.4 Continued

Condition	Presenting signs	Epidemiology	Other significant clinical and laboratory findings	Diagnosis
Upper alimentary tract squamous cell carcinoma	Weight loss. Ruminal tympany. Biphasic diarrhoea	Single animal. Old beef cows, over 8 years. Access to bracken-infested pasture	Poor condition. Normal temperature. High proportion of cases have oral papillomas. Cud-dropping. Faeces have excess of long fibres. May be possible to palpate oropharyngeal tumours	Clinical signs. Access to bracken. Post-mortem findings
Molybdenosis	Profuse diarrhoea begins within a few days of access to suspect pasture. Homogeneous, watery faeces	Group problem. Both dairy and beef cattle. Any age. Geographically well defined areas	Progressive weight loss. Decrease in milk yield. Normal temperature. Signs of secondary copper deficiency. Blood molybdenum values of 0.10 ppm. Hypocupraemia	Clinical signs. Response to copper therapy and, or, removal from suspect pasture

Adult cattle infected with *S. dublin* invariably become life-long persistent carriers of the infection. They excrete the organism in their faeces either continuously or intermittently but especially around parturition, frequently infecting the calf at that time. In contrast, adult cattle infected with *S. typhimurium* or other serotypes cease shedding the organism in a matter of weeks or months (although in some cases this can be as long as 11 months).

Bovine salmonellosis is characterized by a severe haemorrhagic enteritis of sudden onset, with marked depression, decreased appetite, pyrexia, often as high as 41°C (106°F), and a marked reduction in milk yield. Abdominal pain may be a feature and affected animals can pass casts of intestinal mucosa. The condition frequently originates and is most serious in recently calved cows, but an entire herd may suddenly show inappetence with a dramatic drop in milk yield from one milking to the next; other clinical signs developing subsequently.

Notwithstanding this classical description of salmonellosis there are reports in which haemorrhagic enteritis does not occur but where the presenting signs are marked depression, inappetence with hollow empty flanks, agalactia, and only scant, soft faeces. Sick, pyrexic pregnant cows may abort following infection with any *Salmonella* species serotype but abortion may be the first and/or only clinical sign of *S. dublin* infection.

Mortality rates vary but the use of antibiotics will reduce mortality to less than 5 %. Diagnosis is based on the clinical signs, bacteriological examination of faeces and pathological examination of any dead animals. Bacteriological examination of the milk filter sock may be a helpful procedure if salmonellosis is suspected in dairy herds. Serological tests are of little value for diagnosing clinically active disease or for diagnosing retrospectively.

WINTER DYSENTERY

Winter dysentery has been reported from most of the major dairying areas of the world but the prevalence in Britain is unknown.

The exact aetiology has not been determined. For many

years it was suggested that *Campylobacter* (*Vibrio*) *fetus* sub-species *jejuni* was responsible. More recently, viruses, enteroviruses and a coronavirus, have been implicated.

The disease occurs during the winter-housing period, often 2–3 weeks after cows have been housed. It is characterized by a sudden, explosive outbreak of profuse, dark green to black diarrhoea; which on careful examination may contain small spots of blood. The condition rapidly spreads throughout the entire adult milking herd. Accompanying the diarrhoea there is a moderate to severe drop in milk yield. The younger and most recently calved cows are reported to be the most severely affected. Elevated temperatures are rarely found at the time of the diarrhoea, but a low-grade pyrexia, up to 40°C (104°F), is said to precede the diarrhoea by 24–48 h.

Individual animals recover without treatment within 3–4 days and the herd is usually free of the disease in 2–3 weeks. Fatalities are extremely rare.

OVEREATING ACIDOSIS

Access to excessive quantities of highly fermentable carbohydrate foods such as grain or concentrates can produce an acute syndrome within 24–48 h. Affected animals are weak and extremely dull, some may be recumbent and others may have a staggering drunken gait. There is a profuse, sweet-smelling, light-coloured diarrhoea which may contain obvious particles of grain. Ruminal distension accompanied by ruminal statis occurs and the rectal temperature is likely to be subnormal. Tachypnoea and tachycardia are common findings; the higher the heart rate, the poorer the prognosis. Affected animals often appear blind, with a poor or absent eye preservation reflex and a sluggish pupillary reflex.

Examination of the ruminal fluid will reveal an increased acidity, with a pH of less than 5 and motile protozoa will be seen on microscopical examination.

MALIGNANT CATARRHAL FEVER

Malignant catarrhal fever is a rare disease which, although outbreaks have been recorded in cattle in Africa and North

America, is normally only seen as a single animal incident. It tends to occur in young adult cattle and in Europe it frequently occurs in animals which have had close contact with lambing ewes. The clinical disease is never seen in sheep, but deer are highly susceptible to this sheep-associated form of malignant catarrhal fever.

The causal agent of the wildebeest-associated African form of malignant catarrhal fever is a herpesvirus, (bovine herpesvirus 3) but as yet no similar virus has been isolated from the sheep-associated European form of the disease. A survey of a small number of British sheep has shown that many are serologically positive of the wildebeest-associated herpesvirus. Malignant catarrhal fever is an example of a lymphoproliferative disease and the clinical signs arise as a result of a dysfunction of the immune system, in particular the large granular lymphocytes.

Diarrhoea occurs in malignant catarrhal fever, although varying in consistency from scant soft faeces to profuse diarrhoea. However, the other clinical signs tend to be much more dramatic. There is marked depression, anorexia and a persistent pyrexia (40.5–41.5°C [105–106°F]). A copious mucopurulent, oculonasal discharge develops which accumulates around the eyes and rhinarium, with occlusion of the nares often causing respiratory stertor. In addition to the ocular discharge, there is intense scleral congestion and a bilateral corneal opacity which starts at the edge of the sclera and spreads centripetally. Photophobia as a result of an iridocyclitis is also present.

Marked hyperaemia of the oral mucous membranes is a feature, with erosion and diphtheresis of the cheek papillae and palate. The mouth appears to be extremely painful and excess salivation is present. The superficial lymph nodes are invariably enlarged. Haematuria and cystitis with frequent micturition are prominent signs. In addition moist, hyperaemic skin lesions are frequently found in the perineal region and other sites and there is often evidence of an encephalitis.

The disease is invariably fatal with death occurring within 5–10 days of the onset of clinical signs. Diagnosis is based on the clinical signs, the post-mortem examination findings and the vasculitis found histologically. Diffuse bilateral corneal opacity and enlarged lymph nodes are not features of mucosal disease. Early acute photosensitization may be confused with malignant catarrhal fever, but the lesions in the former condition are confined to the white parts of the body and there are no oral lesions.

RAGWORT POISONING

Ragwort (*Senecio jacoboea*) is one of several plants found worldwide which contain hepatotoxic pyrrolizidine alkaloids. The prevalence of ragwort poisoning is low and sporadic. However, if the plant has been ensiled, several cases may occur within a short time. The liver lesions are progressive and irreversible but the clinical signs do not appear until several weeks, even months, after consuming the plant.

In many instances a severe diarrhoea, often black in colour, heralds the onset of this disease. This diarrhoea is accompanied by severe straining and prolapse of the rectum. Affected animals are extremely dull and have a staggering ataxic hindquarter gait. The hind feet tend to be dragged rather than placed when walking. As further evidence of hepatoencephalopathy, head pressing may also be noted. Although the bilirubin levels are frequently elevated, clinical jaundice is often difficult to detect.

The liver is not palpable, but a fluid thrill caused by very oedematous intestines and mesentery may be elicited across the abdomen. Death occurs within a few days. Less severely affected animals may survive for several weeks with weight loss, decreased milk yield, and possibly photosensitization being the main clinical signs.

Laboratory tests to confirm a diagnosis of ragwort poisoning are frequently unrewarding. As noted above, the concentration of bilirubin is increased in many cases but not greatly so. Furthermore although many of the liver-function enzyme tests have raised values in the early (non-clinical) phase of the disease, these values have frequently returned to normal before clinical signs are apparent. Serum enzyme tests which may be useful are alkaline phosphatase, γ-glutamyl transferase and possibly aspartate aminotransferase. The bromsulphthalein clearance test will only give significantly abnormal values when most of the normal liver tissue has been destroyed. There is a hyperammonaemia terminally. Biopsy of the liver may be the most useful diagnostic aid.

Diagnosis is based on the clinical signs, a history of access to ragwort and the laboratory data. At post-mortem examination the liver is reduced in size, and on section, very firm and fibrotic. There is marked visceral oedema, but only small volumes of ascitic fluid. Histology of the liver will reveal typical megalocytes with "bird's eye" nucleoli.

It should be remembered that certain mycotoxins, such as aflatoxins and those produced by the fungus *Phomopsis leptostromiformis*, a contaminant of growing lupins, may produce a similar clinical syndrome also as a result of hepatotoxicity.

ARSENIC POISONING

With the decreasing use of arsenic based products in agriculture, the possibility of arsenic poisoning in farm animals is becoming more remote. However, it must be borne in mind if cattle have had access to old dumps or to organic arsenicals.

There is a delay of 20–48 h between ingestion of the arsenic and the onset of clinical signs which is extremely rapid; death can occur with no premonitory signs. In less acute cases affected animals are depressed, with severe diarrhoea which frequently contains blood and shreds of intestinal epithelium. They often exhibit marked abdominal pain and there is complete anorexia. A tachycardia is present but there is no pyrexia. Death occurs within 12–36 h of the onset of clinical signs.

The less acute cases can resemble salmonellosis but the history of possible access to arsenic compounds and deaths with no premonitory signs should be of assistance.

In the live animal, diagnosis can be confirmed by the detection of arsenic in the urine. In those animals which have died, arsenic concentrations in the liver greater than 10–15 ppm (wet basis) are diagnostic. At post-mortem examination there is a rumenitis with shedding of the mucosa, exposing a congested, haemorrhagic muscular layer. Severe abomasitis and enteritis are also present.

CHRONIC CONDITIONS

JOHNE'S DISEASE (PARATUBERCULOSIS)

Johne's disease, caused by *Mycobacterium paratuberculosis*, is still very common. It affects both dairy and beef animals. The peak age incidence is between 4 and 7 years but clinical disease can occur from 2 to 15 years. Affected animals have a history of weight loss and diarrhoea. Initially the diarrhoea is intermittent but eventually becomes persistent and profuse; the faeces are well comminuted and homogeneous. There is loss of skeletal muscle, especially from the hindquarters (Fig. 16.1).

Once they become clinical cases, dairy cows suffer a dramatic drop in milk yield, but affected cows have frequently had a reduced milk yield in the previous lactation. The calves of affected beef cows tend to be poorly grown for their age. Transient submandibular oedema, which often disappears when the diarrhoea becomes persistent, is present in a small proportion of cases. Loss of coat pigmentation may occur. Until the terminal stages of the disease, the animal remains bright and alert, has a good appetite and ruminates normally.

Examination of the faeces by the method of Cunningham and Gilmour (1959) will reveal clumps of acid-fast organisms morphologically resembling *M. paratuberculosis* in about 50 % of cases at the first examination, but negative findings do not

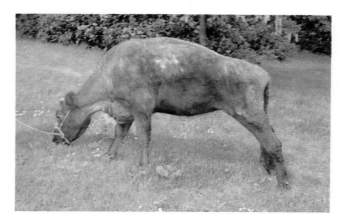

Fig. 16.1
Typical case of
Johne's disease.

preclude the disease. Serological tests are of extremely limited value although 90 % of clinical cases will give a positive complement fixation reaction. Culture of *M. paratuberculosis* from faeces is too time consuming for confirmation of clinical cases, as cultures require to be incubated for up to 3 months before they can be discarded as negative. However, it is likely to prove the most useful method of detecting preclinical cases.

Diagnosis is based on characteristic clinical signs and, if present, clumps of typical acid-fast organisms in the faeces will confirm the disease. Where necessary the diagnosis should be confirmed by post-mortem examination and histological examination of the intestine.

MUCOSAL DISEASE

Mucosal disease, caused by mucosal disease/bovine virus diarrhoea virus is most commonly seen in animals less than 2 years old. It can occur in adult cattle, usually those less than 4 years old, as sporadic, single-case incidents.

Clinically affected animals are depressed with a reduced appetite and a history of weight loss. The diarrhoea is almost always continuous but can sometimes be intermittent. Frequently excess saliva is present around the lips and muzzle. Examination of the mouth reveals hyperaemic mucous membranes and numerous small irregular erosions on the dental pad and the hard and soft palates. Linear cracks and fissures, some with diphtheresis (Fig. 16.2), are found at the

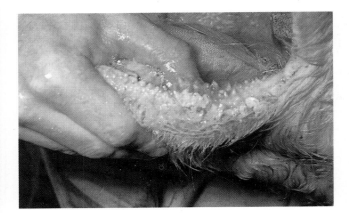

Fig. 16.2
Mucosal disease: ulcers and diphtheresis at commissures of lips.

comissures of the lips but these may not be present in very acute cases. Ulceration of the dorsum of the tongue is uncommon, but when it does occur the ulcers are deeper than those seen elsewhere in the mouth. In addition, hyperkeratinization at the skin/rhinarium junction (Fig. 16.3), congestion of the conjunctival mucosae and a moderate mucopurulent ocular discharge are common.

Lameness with ulceration of the interdigital clefts of all four feet accompanied by hyperaemia and a hyperkeratinization of the posterior aspects of the pasterns occurs. In a minority of cases there is superficial necrosis of the skin, especially in the groin and axillae. Small raised lesions may also be detected in the perineal region.

Diagnosis is based on clinical signs and can be confirmed by virus isolation, serology and post-mortem examination.

OSTERTAGIASIS

Ostertagiasis as a result of infection with *Ostertagia ostertagi* is more prevalent in immature cattle. However, both Type 1 and Type 2 ostertagiasis can be severe and debilitating conditions in adult cattle. Both susceptible dairy and beef animals may be affected. They require to have ingested pasture carrying fairly heavy burdens of *O. ostertagi* L3 larvae. This most commonly occurs when dairy cows graze pasture which has been contaminated by immature animals earlier in the

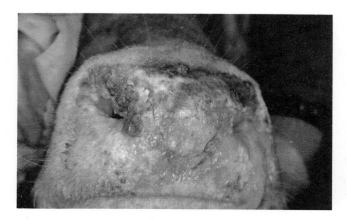

Fig. 16.3
Mucosal disease: rhinarium.

grazing season. In beef cows it can arise through the overgrazing of improved pastures which have become heavily contaminated. Type 1 ostertagiasis occurs in the autumn and Type 2 disease occurs in the spring or early summer following a period of inhibited larval development.

Clinically, ill thrift, weight loss and a profuse homogeneous diarrhoea are seen in a group of animals, possibly the whole herd or at least a group within the herd which has had a similar grazing history. A significant decrease in milk yield occurs in dairy cows. Subcutaneous oedema may be noted especially in Type 2 ostertagiasis.

As a result of the damage to the abomasal mucosa, serum concentrations of pepsinogen are increased. In overt clinical disease the serum pepsinogen values will be in excess of 3000 miu of tyrosine. Hypoalbuminaemia also occurs. Faecal trichostrongyle egg counts are higher in Type 1 disease than in Type 2 ostertagiasis.

Diagnosis is based on careful consideration of the clinical signs, the grazing history and the seasonal factors which influence this disease. The serum pepsinogen test is an extremely useful diagnostic tool. Pathological examination together with parasitological examination of the abomasum for total burdens of *O. ostertagi* will give confirmation if necessary.

Occasionally, ostertagiasis may occur in a single animal, which for some reason has been managed differently, for example, beef bulls kept in small paddocks out of the breeding season. In these instances clinical differentiation from Johne's disease can be quite difficult. Grazing history and laboratory tests should enable a correct diagnosis to be made. The clinical response to any of the modern anthelmintics may prove rewarding, especially in Type 1 ostertagiasis.

RENAL AMYLOIDOSIS

Renal amyloidosis is a rare condition caused by the deposition of amyloid in the kidneys resulting in a nephrotic syndrome. It is most frequently seen in middle-aged dairy cows in which it occurs as primary amyloidosis. Amyloid deposition secondary to chronic septic foci also occurs and in this form of the disease any type or age of animal can be affected.

In primary renal amyloidosis, affected animals are usually in good condition. There is marked subcutaneous submandibular, presternal and ventral oedema, and a profuse, homogeneous watery diarrhoea. On rectal examination a greatly enlarged left kidney will be palpated. Urine analysis will reveal a marked proteinuria, with values in excess of 300 mg/dl of urine and often more than 1000 mg/dl. As a result of this protein loss, a severe hypoalbuminaemia is present with values as low as 10 g/litre or less. Raised plasma urea values are also found.

Affected cows usually become recumbent within two to three weeks of first being presented and have to be destroyed. At post mortem examination the greatly enlarged, two to three times normal size, pale, yellowish-brown waxy kidneys are almost pathognomonic (Fig. 16.4). In addition to the subcutaneous oedema, there is marked visceral oedema.

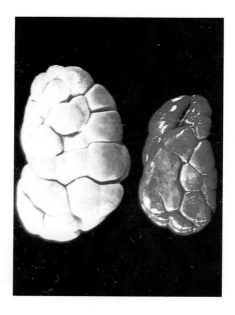

Fig. 16.4
Renal amyloidosis: affected kidney and kidney from another animal of similar size.

SQUAMOUS CELL CARCINOMA OF THE UPPER ALIMENTARY TRACT

A high incidence area of squamous cell carcinoma of the upper alimentary tract, affecting the stratified squamous epithelium of the mouth, pharynx, oesophagus and forestomachs has been identified in Scotland and north east England. These tumours appear to be associated with grazing marginal land infested with bracken, *Pteridium aquilinum*. For this reason the syndrome is almost exclusively seen in adult beef cows and almost every case is more than 8 years old.

The tumours are found at three main sites, the oropharynx, the oesophagus and the rumen (Fig. 16.5) where they can involve the ruminal wall, the cardia, the reticular groove and the distal oesophagus. The presenting signs depend upon the location of the tumours, but weight loss, diarrhoea and ruminal tympany are those most commonly noted. In contrast to the homogeneous diarrhoea of Johne's disease, the diarrhoea in this syndrome is often biphasic with a fibrous component of solid ingesta and a fluid, water component. Food is poorly comminuted and the proportion of fibres more than 2 cm long

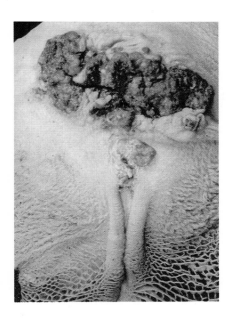

Fig. 16.5
Upper alimentary squamous cell carcinoma: tumour in rumen.

in the faeces is greatly increased. If the lesion is in the oropharynx, the cow may drool saliva, with halitosis and, or, respiratory stertor. Ruminal tympany may be present when tumours are located in either the oesophagus or the rumen. This tympany is seldom severe or life threatening, but the strength and frequency of ruminal contractions are reduced. The majority of cases have small, glistening, while papillomas caused by bovine papilloma virus on the posterior hard and soft palates. These are frequently more easily palpated than seen. The regurgitation of boluses of food (cud dropping) is a common finding in this syndrome.

Pathologically the tumours are variable in size; those in the rumen may be up to 50 cm in diameter. There are two main forms, either raised cauliflower-like masses or ulcerative plaques. Both have a brown surface covered with a foul smelling friable detritus. Metastasis occurs in about 40 % of cases. Microscopically the malignant squamous cells are arranged in groups or in cords frequently with marked keratinization.

Diagnosis is based on the epidemiology, the clinical syndrome and the characteristic pathological findings.

Occasionally, the biphasic diarrhoea described above is seen in old beef cows with very worn and, or, missing molar teeth. Weight loss is also associated with this syndrome.

OTHER ALIMENTARY TUMOURS

Other alimentary tumours such as alimentary lymphosarcoma and abomasal adenocarcinoma are extremely rare. They present as cases of chronic intractable diarrhoea with weight loss. Pathological examination is required for diagnosis.

All bovine tumours or suspect tumours, excluding papillomas, haemangiomas and haemangiosarcomas are notifiable under the Enzootic Bovine Leukosis Order (1977).

ABDOMINAL FAT NECROSIS

Sporadic cases of fat necrosis are occasionally identified on routine rectal examination of the reproductive tract. The hard, firm, knobbly masses of necrotic fat are frequently benign, but can cause several syndromes, depending on their location, one of which is profuse diarrhoea and weight loss. The condition has been associated with the Channel Island breeds, but can occur in herds in which the cows are kept in very good condition, or individual show animals. Affected animals are usually middle-aged to old. If the firm, often almost bone-like masses cannot be felt on rectal examination, clinical diagnosis is very difficult, and even if they are palpated, something more serious like a tumour is frequently suspected.

MOLYBDENOSIS

This condition, characterized by persistent diarrhoea, decreased milk yield, weight loss and poor coat, occurs when cattle graze pastures on molybdenum-rich soils. Such geologically defined areas (e.g. the "Teart" pastures of Somerset) are likely to have been well recognized and preventative measures instituted. Other signs such as lameness, stiffness and achromotrichia owing to secondary copper deficiency have also been noted. However, the possibility of molybdenum pollution of pasture from industrial plants which may give rise to the syndrome in unexpected locations should be borne in mind.

PLANT POISONING

Some plants, including ragwort, which have been associated with diarrhoea in adult cattle are shown in Table 16.5. Animals affected by acute bracken poisoning frequently have diarrhoea which contains frank blood, but in addition to the pyrexia there is pallor and petechiation of the mucous membranes. Oak poisoning can also cause a haemorrhagic diarrhoea, but

Table 16.5 Diarrhoea in adult cattle: Plant poisonings.

Bracken (acute bracken poisoning)	
Castor seed residue	Hound's tongue
Fodder beet	Oak
Hemlock	Ragwort

the toxic nephropathy which occurs in this syndrome is much more significant both clinically and pathologically.

REFERENCES AND FURTHER READING

Brownlie, J. (1985). *Veterinary Record* Supplement *In Practice* **7**, 195.
Chiodini, R. J., Van Kruiningen, H. J. & Merkal, R. S. (1984). *Cornell Veterinarian* **74**, 218.
Clegg, F. G., Chiejina, S. N., Duncan, A. L., Kay, R. N. & Wray, C. (1983). *Veterinary Record* **112**, 580.
Cunningham, M. P. & Gilmour, N. J. L. (1959). *Veterinary Record* **71**, 47.
Davies, D. C. & Jebbett, I. H. (1981). *Veterinary Record* Supplement *In Practice* **3**, 14.
Duffell, S. J. & Harkness, J. W. (1985). *Veterinary Record* **117**, 240.
Gilmour, N. J. L. (1976). *Veterinary Record* **99**, 433.
Hinton, M. (1974). *British Veterinary Journal* **130**, 556.
Jarrett, W. F. H., McNeil, P. E., Grimshaw, W. T. R., Selman, I. E. & McIntyre, W. I. M. (1978). *Nature* **274**, 215.
Petrie, L., Armour, J. & Stevenson, S. H. (1984). *Veterinary Record* **114**, 168.
Reid, H. W., Buxton, D., Berrie, E., Pow, I. & Finlayson, J. (1984). *Veterinary Record* **114**, 582.
Richardson, A. (1975). *Journal of Hygiene (Cambridge)* **74**, 195.
Rossiter, P. B. (1981). *Journal of Comparative Pathology* **91**, 303.
Selman, I. E., Reid, J. F. S., Armour, J. & Jennings, F. W. (1976). *Veterinary Record* **99**, 141.
Selman, I. E., Wiseman, A., Murray, M. & Wright, N. G. (1974). *Veterinary Record* **94**, 483.
Tutt, J. B. & Hoare, D. I. B. (1974). *Veterinary Record* **95**, 334.

CHAPTER 17

Clinical Aspects of the Bovine Virus Diarrhoea/Mucosal Disease Complex in Cattle

JOE BROWNLIE

INTRODUCTION

Cattle infected with bovine virus diarrhoea (BVD) virus can present a variety of clinical signs, both enteric and respiratory. It was this variety that led originally to the description of two separate diseases, bovine virus diarrhoea and mucosal disease of cattle. Both diseases are now thought to be caused by the same virus.

Furthermore, as the virus is widespread throughout the national herd there is every opportunity for infection. Most adult cattle have antibodies to BVD virus by the age of 2 years. However, there now appears to be a significant number of "closed" herds with no detectable antibody to the virus; these represent particularly susceptible groups of cattle.

BOVINE VIRUS DIARRHOEA VIRUS

BVD virus is an RNA virus which, with border disease virus and hog cholera virus, forms a group which is classified as

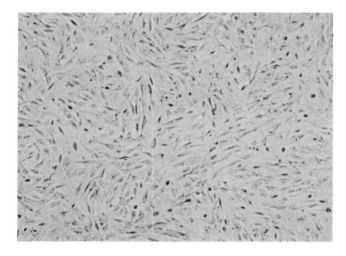

Fig. 17.1
Monolayer of calf
testis cells infected
with non-cytopathic
BVD virus (courtesy
of M. C. Clarke,
IRAD, Compton).

the pestiviruses in the Togaviridae. The three viruses cross-
react antigenically and have other biological and structural
similarities.

Although isolates of BVD virus from different clinical cases
of disease may be serologically distinguishable, the most
obvious difference is their separation into one of two forms
by their growth characteristics in cell culture: they may
be non-cytopathic (Fig. 17.1) or cytopathic (Fig. 17.2). This

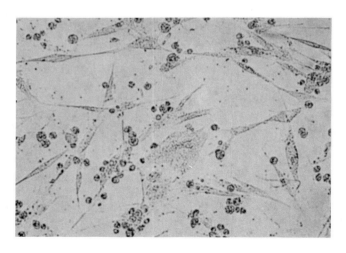

Fig. 17.2
Monolayer of calf
testis cells infected
with cytopathic BVD
virus. Note rounded
and vacuolated cells
with cell depletion
(courtesy of M. C.
Clarke, IRAD,
Compton).

distinction has only recently been shown to be important in the aetiology of mucosal disease.

AETIOLOGY OF MUCOSAL DISEASE

An explanation for the aetiology of mucosal disease has recently been put forward which proposes that mucosal disease develops following an early *in utero* infection with non-cytopathic BVD virus resulting in the birth of a calf with a persistent viraemia. If this calf is later superinfected with a cytopathic BVD virus, mucosal disease can develop (Fig. 17.3).

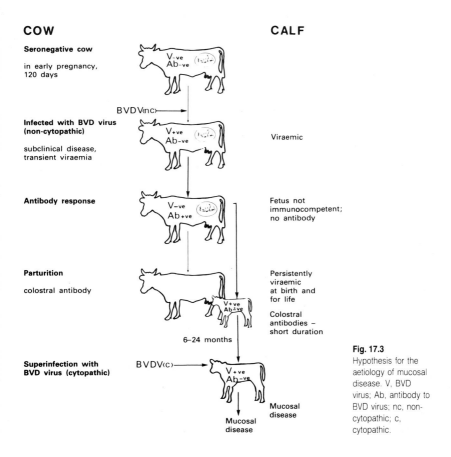

COW

Seronegative cow

in early pregnancy, 120 days

BVDV(nc)⟶

Infected with BVD virus (non-cytopathic)

subclinical disease, transient viraemia

Antibody response

Parturition

colostral antibody

6–24 months

Superinfection with BVD virus (cytopathic)

BVDV(c)⟶

Mucosal disease

CALF

Viraemic

Fetus not immunocompetent; no antibody

Persistently viraemic at birth and for life

Colostral antibodies – short duration

Mucosal disease

Fig. 17.3 Hypothesis for the aetiology of mucosal disease. V, BVD virus; Ab, antibody to BVD virus; nc, non-cytopathic; c, cytopathic.

It is only those animals that are persistently infected with non-cytopathic BVD virus which will later develop mucosal disease.

ASPECTS OF INFECTION WITH BVD VIRUS

ACUTE INFECTION

BVD disease refers to the acute infection of seronegative cattle with BVD virus. The original description of explosive outbreaks of diarrhoea caused by the virus is now rarely observed and most infections may be subclinical. Experimental infection of calves produces a similarly mild disease with a transient leucopenia and some animals may show a rise in temperature. In both natural and experimental infections antibodies are produced in 2–3 weeks and the animal appears immune to later challenge.

IN UTERO INFECTION

Crucial to the development of mucosal disease is the *in utero* infection of the fetus with non-cytopathic BVD virus. There is no evidence from either field or experimental work that persistent viraemia occurs with cytopathic BVD virus.

Infection with non-cytopathic BVD virus must be before 120 days of gestation for the virus to persist. The immune system is not functionally developed before that stage so the virus can become widely established in the fetal tissue. Subsequently although the immune system is competent it recognizes the virus as "self" and a state of immune tolerance develops. This tolerance allows the non-cytopathic virus to persist into neonatal life and also the unchecked replication of superinfecting cytopathic BVD virus.

ABORTIONS AND STILLBIRTHS

A feature of BVD virus infection in pregnant cattle is the frequency of abortions and stillbirths. Retrospective inquiries following a mucosal disease outbreak will often reveal a series of abortions and births of dead or weak calves. Sometimes there may have been an infertility problem with increased return to service caused by early embryonic loss.

CONGENITAL ABNORMALITIES

Fetopathology caused by BVD virus infection has been well documented. Typical is the intrauterine growth retardation observed in various organs, e.g. thymus, and also the pathology caused to the central nervous system. Clinically, affected calves are born weak, ataxic and often with visual disorders. They may have antibody to BVD virus and no virus.

MIXED INFECTIONS WITH BVD VIRUS AND OTHER PATHOGENS

BVD virus is considered to be an immunosuppressive agent which infects the cells of the immune system, resulting in leucopenia. There is a reduction in the defence mechanisms and as a result the host is more susceptible to infection with other pathogens. Such mixed infections have been reported from both field and experimental work and may represent an important sequel of acute BVD virus infection.

For example, a combined experimental infection with BVD virus and *Pasteurella haemolytica* results in a severe fibrinopurulent bronchopneumonia with the area of pneumonic lesions increasing to 40–75 % compared with 5–15 % with pasteurella alone. This synergism has also been observed with parainfluenza, infectious bovine rhinotracheitis and respiratory syncytial viruses.

MUCOSAL DISEASE

CLINICAL SIGNS

Mucosal disease usually occurs in 6–24-month-old cattle and is invariably fatal. The cattle possess no specific antibodies to the infecting virus even though it has persisted in the blood during their lifetime.

The first clinical sign is usually anorexia. Close inspection may reveal erosions either on the oral mucosa particularly at the gingival margin (Figure 17.4), on the tongue (Fig. 17.5), the external nares and in the buccal and nasal cavities. These lesions are present in about 75 % of cases. In some animals, there is desquamation of the muzzle with extensive crusting and even purulent exudate. There may also be nasal discharge (Figure 17.4).

Lesions can be seen around the coronet and on the interdigital surface, often with redness and swelling. The animal is disinclined to walk and soon becomes recumbent. There is often profuse diarrhoea and invariably death. Death can be so sudden that it may be the first clinical sign, but normally it follows 3–10 days from the onset of symptoms.

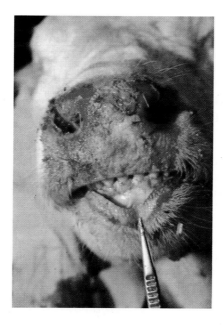

Fig. 17.4
Muzzle of calf with mucosal disease. Note the desquamation and crusting. At the gingival margin there is hyperaemia and mucosal erosions.

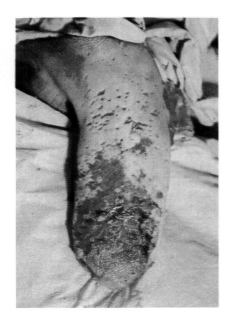

Fig. 17.5
Tongue of a calf with mucosal disease showing
complete loss of epithelium on the apex.

POST-MORTEM FINDINGS

Much useful information can be gained from a detailed post-mortem examination of suspected cases of mucosal disease. The full extent of oral, lingual and buccal erosions should be observed. A common finding in the buccal mucosa is that the small erosions have coalesced into larger areas of necrosis and sloughed epithelium.

Similar erosions may be seen in the oesophagus. Ruminal lesions, if present, are areas of congestion and oedema along the ruminal pillars. Ulceration is rare. The large ruminal papillae can be reduced in size.

The abomasum and small intestine provide the most reliable sites for inspection but immediate autopsy is important as post-mortem changes in the gut are rapid and gaseous extension can often mask the enteric erosions.

The abomasum usually shows several (5–50) small discoid erosions, about 5 mm diameter, with surrounding hyperaemia in the mucosa. Submucosal petechial haemorrhages are a

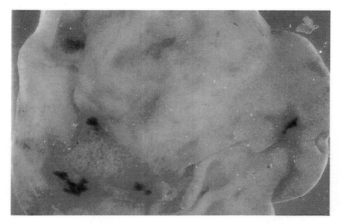

Fig. 17.6
Post-mortem
appearance of the
abomasum with
erosions surrounded
by congestion and
petechial
haemorrhage.

common finding, particularly in the pylorus (Fig. 17.6). Occasionally, the erosions can be larger and ulcerated.

The small intestine, if opened throughout its length to expose the antimesenteric surface, will reveal oval erosions (2–5 cm long) that overlie the lymphatic tissue in Peyer's patches. The erosions may vary from 2–3 to 30–40. Towards the terminal ileum the erosions can become extensive and may be up to 10–20 cm in length. The exposed submucosal surface of the erosions can vary from the chronic lesion, with food adhering (Fig. 17.7), to the acutely congested one often with interluminal haemorrhage.

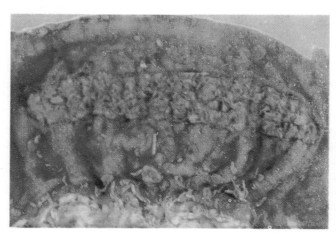

Fig. 17.7
Mucosal disease.
Post-mortem
appearance of the
small intestine. Some
erosions may appear
chronic, even with
food adhering to the
surface.

In the large bowel, there may be congestion of the mucosa which gives a thickening to the mucosal folds and a striped appearance. There may also occasionally be petechial haemorrhages and small erosions along the folds. The contents are dark, watery and often foul smelling.

FIELD OUTBREAKS

A number of mucosal disease outbreaks have been extensively investigated and several salient features have become recognized:

(1) The initial investigation is usually prompted following the rapid deterioration or perhaps death of an animal in the 6–24-month-old age group.
(2) The clinical investigation, together with post-mortem findings, guides the practitioner to consider a diagnosis of mucosal disease.
(3) Examination of blood samples from the remaining animals in the group reveals a number that have little or no antibody to BVD virus and some that are also viraemic.

It is therefore essential to examine all in-contact animals for the presence of both virus and antibody. There are four possible categories for these animals (Fig. 17.8). Within these four combinations, it is only animals in category 4(b) and occasional animals in category 3(b) that will subsequently develop mucosal disease. The early identification of these animals is all important.

SEQUENTIAL STUDY OF AN OUTBREAK

Most of the larger outbreaks of mucosal disease that have been studied have shown that, at some time, new animals have been introduced into a "closed" unit or herd of susceptible cattle, often about 18 months previously.

The newly introduced animal can bring in the virus either as an acute infection or as a persistent one. The virus is then transmitted by animal-to-animal contact. If seronegative heifers in early pregnancy are present, there is a basis for *in*

Category	Animal	Status	Result of exposure to BVD virus	Final antibody status
1	V − ve Ab − ve	no previous exposure to BVD virus	transient mild infection	+ve
2	V − ve Ab + ve	previous exposure to BVD virus from 120 days gestation onwards	immune	+ve

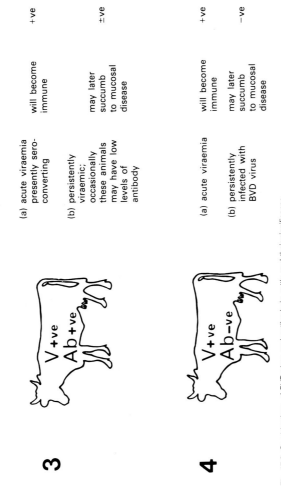

3

V +ve
Ab +ve

(a) acute viraemia presently sero-converting — will become immune — +ve

(b) persistently viraemic; occasionally these animals may have low levels of antibody — may later succumb to mucosal disease — ±ve

4

V +ve
Ab −ve

(a) acute viraemia — will become immune — +ve

(b) persistently infected with BVD virus — may later succumb to mucosal disease — −ve

Fig. 17.8 Combinations of BVD virus and antibody in cattle and their significance.

utero infection, with the subsequent production of persistently viraemic calves and later an outbreak of mucosal disease. Obviously, should the introduced animal be persistently infected, there is far greater chance for transmission of virus to susceptible cattle. At present there is little evidence for BVD virus becoming latent following acute infection and at a later date being able to recrudesce.

Once a case of mucosal disease has been diagnosed, the presence of cytopathic virus can be assumed. The transmission of cytopathic BVD virus is rapid and, once super-infected, persistently infected cattle rapidly lose condition and invariably die.

An analysis of all the effects that can follow from BVD virus infection reveals the extent and true cost of an outbreak (Fig. 17.9). By the time the practitioner is called, the earlier damage caused by virus infection has already occurred, but has not been associated with BVD virus.

CONTROL MEASURES

To prevent an outbreak

In the UK there is no effective vaccine and caution will be needed before live virus vaccines are introduced. Reports from Europe and the USA have shown that live vaccines which originate from cytopathic BVD virus can precipitate mucosal disease.

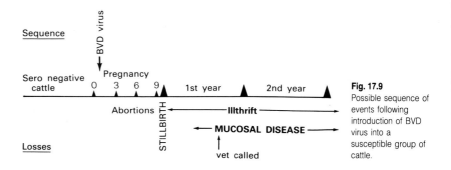

Fig. 17.9 Possible sequence of events following introduction of BVD virus into a susceptible group of cattle.

The best means of control at present is to screen newly introduced stock for the presence of virus and antibody. This is particularly important for new animals that will be in contact with pregnant cattle, i.e. a new bull or young heifer.

During an outbreak

The remaining animals in the susceptible group should be bled and examined for BVD virus and antibody. Any animal found to be persistently viraemic should be either isolated or, as experience now indicates, sent for immediate slaughter.

Isolation to prevent contact with cytopathic virus can occasionally work, but by the time the laboratory diagnosis can be made, there has been general transmission of cytopathic virus throughout the remaining cattle. Cattle can quickly lose condition following superinfection and there is little remaining carcass value.

DIFFERENTIAL DIAGNOSIS

BOVINE VIRUS DIARRHOEA

A primary BVD virus infection is usually mild and rarely diagnosed except by serology.

MUCOSAL DISEASE

There are three major features of mucosal disease that may be present: mucosal erosions, diarrhoea and death. The differential diagnosis should be as described below.

Foot-and-mouth disease

All cloven-hooved animals are susceptible to foot-and-mouth disease which is characterized by pyrexia, anorexia and excessive salivation. Tongue and buccal erosions are consistently present and are preceded by the formation and rupture of vesicles containing straw-coloured fluid. This contrasts with mucosal disease where the erosions arise not from vesicles but directly from necrosis of erythematous areas in the mucosa.

With foot-and-mouth disease the morbidity can be 100 % whereas mortality is less than 5 % in adults, although it may rise to 50 % in younger animals. With mucosal disease the morbidity of a herd is lower and generally restricted to the 6–24-month age groups, but mortality may approach 100 %.

Malignant catarrhal fever

Malignant catarrhal fever is another disease characterized by gastroenteritis and an erosive stomatitis. There is usually bilateral corneal opacity and general lymph node enlargement. The serosa of the abomasum and large intestine is hyperaemic, oedematous and often with haemorrhage into the rumen.

The small intestine shows less damage and the discrete ulceration of Peyer's patches, seen in mucosal disease, is not present. Sporadic cases of malignant catarrhal fever are seen in the UK and diagnosis depends on histological examination of tissue and cerebrospinal fluid.

Salmonellosis

Salmonellosis is often considered in the differential diagnosis. Outbreaks of acute diarrhoea with some deaths are features common to salmonellosis and mucosal disease. There are rarely oral or intestinal erosions with salmonellosis and often younger calves are more severely affected.

There is frequently a marked spleen, liver and lymph-node enlargement. Diagnosis depends on isolation of bacteria from faeces or post-mortem tissue samples.

Rinderpest

Rinderpest is another disease where vesicles precede erosions on the tongue, oral mucosa, teats and coronet. There is more severe lymph node and intestinal oedema than in mucosal disease but similar Peyer's patch erosions are seen. The morbidity and mortality are both high.

Ibaraki disease

This disease, not yet reported in the UK, is caused by an orbivirus and has been classified as epizootic haemorrhagic disease virus, type V. It presents an erosive stomatitis, abomasitis and often diarrhoea.

There is damage to the oesophageal musculature often resulting in megaoesophagus with the retention of imbibed fluids. These are regurgitated as copious clear mucus fluid through the mouth and sometimes nose. This "deglutative disorder" is particularly characteristic of Ibaraki disease and not seen in mucosal disease. The erosions of Peyer's patches are rarely presented. It is dependent on insect transmission and therefore seasonal.

LABORATORY TECHNIQUES FOR DIAGNOSIS OF BVD VIRUS

DETECTION OF ANTIBODY

Serum neutralization

Serum neutralization depends on the ability of antibodies in the serum to neutralize BVD virus and thereby prevent infection of cell culture. The test usually takes 4–7 days to obtain a result but is dependent on cell-culture facilities and an experienced observer.

ELISA

An enzyme-linked immunosorbent assay (ELISA) technique for BVD virus antibodies that depends on binding of antibody to specific BVD virus antigen has been developed. The test takes 1 day. It requires purified ingredients but is simple to operate and the results can, if necessary, be recorded by eye.

DETECTION OF VIRUS

Cell culture

BVD virus can be cultivated in cell culture monolayers (e.g. calf testis or calf kidney). The cytopathic virus is identified by changes in the monolayers such as vacuolation of cell cytoplasm, rounding of cells and their subsequent lysis. Non-cytopathic virus produces no such changes. Both viruses can be visualized by fluorescein-coupled antibody (Fig. 17.10). Primary identification of these viruses may be made in about 7 days.

a

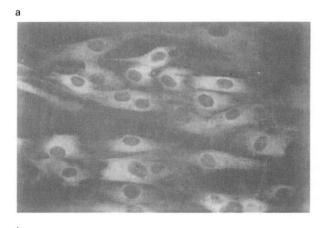

b

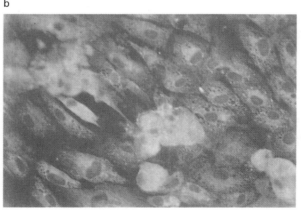

Fig. 17.10
Cell culture monolayers infected with (a) non-cytopathic and (b) cytopathic BVD virus, stained with specific BVD virus fluorescein-coupled antibody.

Enzyme staining

Virus grown on cell-culture monolayers in microtitre assay plates or small petri dishes can be identified by enzyme-linked antibody. This assay may take only 3–4 days.

DEER AND SHEEP

Deer and sheep can be infected by BVD virus. Therefore possible transmission to or from both species should be considered during any outbreak of mucosal disease of cattle.

CONCLUSION

Our understanding of this disease, first described in 1946, has advanced recently and more may be revealed in the next 5 years, so this report should be regarded only as an up-to-date reference. New technology has improved diagnosis of the disease, e.g. ELISA techniques, molecular virology and detailed immunology. There is greater confidence in predicting the course of a disease and in ascribing a correct viral and antibody status to an animal.

It may be suggested that a test for persistent viraemia should be considered in any health inspection of cattle by the practitioner. What is becoming clear is that outbreaks of clinical disease can be the cause of severe loss and that the cattle practitioner needs to be aware of all its aspects.

FURTHER READING

Allison, C. J. (1984). *Veterinary Record* **115**, 110.
Barlow, R. M., Gardiner, A. C. & Nettleton, P. F. (1983). *Journal of Comparative Pathology* **93**, 451.
Brownlie, J., Clarke, M. C. & Howard, C. J. (1984). *Veterinary Record* **114**, 535.
Brownlie, J., Clarke, M. C. & Howard, C. J. (1984). *Veterinary Record* **115**, 158.

Howard, C. J., Clarke, M. C. & Brownlie, J. (1985). *Veterinary Microbiology* **10**, 359.

Nagele, M. J. (1984). *Veterinary Record* **115**, 496.

Roeder, P. L. & Drew, T. W. (1984). *Veterinary Record* **114**, 309.

Control

CHAPTER 18

Feeding Colostrum to Calves

DAVID WHITE

INTRODUCTION

The beneficial effects of feeding colostrum to calves have been suspected for more than 80 years. Despite this, approximately half of all calves sold in the UK have inadequate circulating antibodies.

IMMUNOGLOBINS

Bovine colostrum varies in its constituents from cow to cow and with time of collection with regard to onset of lactation.

There are three main types of immunoglobulins: IgG, IgM and IgA. The IgG class is heterogeneous and can be further subdivided into IgG_1 and IgG_2. IgG is the major immunoglobulin in the sera of adult cattle. In first milk colostrum IgG_1 accounts for 81 % of all antibodies. IgG_2, IgM and IgA make up the rest. IgG_1 is actively concentrated in the colostrum, depleting maternal serum by some 50 % in the final 5 weeks of pregnancy. There is 3–12-fold difference in IgG_1 concentration between colostrum and serum at the end of pregnancy.

Table 18.1 Patency (calves) for different types of immunoglobulin.

Patency (calves)		
	IgM	16 h
	IgA	22 h
	IgG	27 h

PATENCY

The period when the colostral proteins can be absorbed from the small intestine (patency) varies between animals, class of immunoglobulin and method of measurement (Table 18.1). The figures in Table 18.1 represent the average age of the calf when no more antibody will be absorbed from the small intestine. The efficiency of absorption decreases from birth at a variable rate so some calves may not be able to absorb measurable quantities of IgG after 12 h.

The volume of colostrum a cow produces varies between breeds, parity and plane of nutrition. Shortly after birth, even before the calf is able to stand normally, the suck reflex is very strong and a calf will suck to satiation in about 25–30 min, ingesting approximately 7 % of its bodyweight. A second feed increases the efficiency of absorption of the first feed and about 12 h later the calf will suck approximately half the volume of the first feed.

The final concentration of immunoglobulin in the sera of young calves is therefore influenced by the quality of the colostrum (Figs 18.1 and 18.2), how quickly the calf gets it (Figs 18.3 and 18.4) and the quantity ingested. The quality of

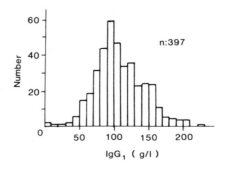

Fig. 18.1
Variation in IgG_1 concentration in first-milk colostrum.

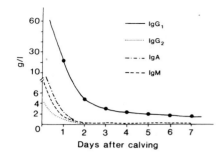

Fig. 18.2
Concentration change in the immunoglobulins of colostrum in the week following parturition.

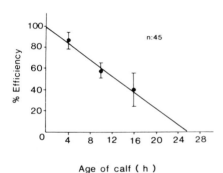

Fig. 18.3
Efficiency of absorption decreases with time.

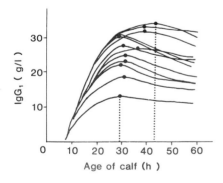

Fig. 18.4
Variation in IgG$_1$ absorbed and time of closure for 12 calves under standard conditions.

colostrum produced and the speed and quantity a calf receives depends on a variety of factors (Table 18.2).

IMPROVING ANTIBODY STATUS OF CALVES

Recommendations to a breeder to improve antibody status of calves include the following:

(1)   At least a 5-week dry period.
(2)   Calve cows in a large loose box with non-slip floor or in open field or paddock away from other cows.
(3)   Maintain plane of nutrition – body condition score 3 – for the last 5 weeks of pregnancy, especially in non-dairy types. Use fish meal or soya-based protein if necessary.
(4)   Ensure each calf receives sufficient colostrum – 6 pints (3.4 l) in the first 6 h is an easy-to-remember working maxim. For a typical Friesian calf (45 kg) this is 7 % of its body weight and it will take 25–30 min to drink it. A second feed to ensure

Table 18.2   Factors affecting colostrum production and the speed and quantity the calf receives.

Colostrum quality decreases with

Foremilking	Short dry period
Subsequent milkings	Immaturity
Mastitis	Immunological naivety

The speed at which a calf receives colostrum

Decreases with:	Dystocia/milk fever/other diseases
	Poor udder conformation
	Poor teat conformation
	Distractions (other cows, calves)
	Slippery floors
	Rough terrain
Increases with:	Good stockmanship
	Calf vitality
	Strong mothering instincts

Quantity of colostrum a calf receives depends on

Breed of dam	Stockmanship
Parity of dam	Calf vitality
Plane of nutrition	Mothering instincts
Husbandry system	

it receives 10 % of its bodyweight in total by 12 h after birth is sufficient for most calves.
(5)   Do not use foremilk unless absolutely necessary.
(6)   Supplement nature if there is any doubt that the calf has received sufficient quantity of quality colostrum quickly.
(7)   Check parturient cows at least every 4 h.
(8)   Following parturition check udder – try each quarter.
(9)   Following dystocia/milk fever, feed calf via oesophageal feeder, bucket or, best of all, a bottle and teat.
(10)   Use stored colostrum – store frozen in 1.5 l packs – using plastic bags or empty ice-cream cartons. Thaw out fully using a warm water bath – some microwave ovens may be suitable but most will overheat parts of the colostrum, denaturing some of the proteins.
(11)   Supplement the dam's supply in mastitic, debilitated and primiparous cows (which may be poor mothers) from frozen stores.
(12)   Only freeze colostrum from the first milking of non-mastic second and third calving, fully vaccinated, healthy cows.
(13)   Don't mix first milk colostrum with colostrum from subsequent milkings.

All of the above consider circulating antibody concentrations. There is evidence to suggest that fed colostrum has a protective effect which can act locally within the gut against a number of viral enteropathogens. This protective effect lasts long after closure (the end of patency). This benefit can be harnessed by using colostrum and milk the cow produces in the second to eighth milkings to feed the calf. The colostrum need not be frozen – no preservative is necessary – and can be fed cold. It is more palatable if fed warm but if it is stored for a long time (10 days) it will clot when warmed up. Palatability of fermenting stored colostrum can be improved by adding sodium bicarbonate.

CHAPTER 19

Control of Tick-borne Disease in Cattle

MIKE VAUGHAN

INTRODUCTION

Four species of tick commonly infest cattle in Great Britain, however, *Ixodes ricinus* (Fig. 19.1) is the only species with importance in disease transmission. The geographical distribution of the four species is as follows:

Dermacentor reticulatus in south west England and Wales.

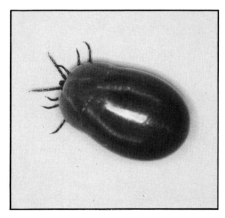

Fig. 19.1
Ixodes ricinus.

Haemaphysalis punctata in limited areas of Kent and Wales.
Ixodes hexagonus all over Britain.
Ixodes ricinus all over Britain.

DISTRIBUTION

Distribution of ticks is dependent upon the existence of suitable habitats which provide a ground layer which is permanently moist (Reid, 1987). These are present in permanent pastures, particularly of the rough grazing type, situated in areas of high rainfall. Cattle must also be present in suitable numbers and Fig. 19.2 below superimposes cattle population figures on tick distribution in England and Wales. Enzootic disease may therefore be expected in certain well defined and separated areas (south west England, parts of Wales and Cumbria and the Scottish Borders).

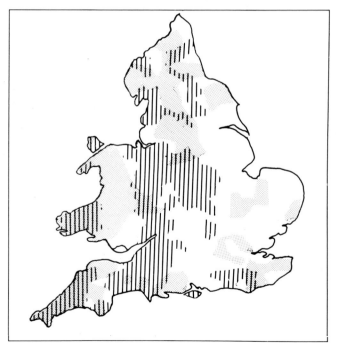

Fig. 19.2
Relative distribution of cattle and ticks in England and Wales. Shaded areas indicate probable limits of tick distribution. Striped areas indicate regions with more than 30 head of cattle per 100 acres (Crown copyright).

LIFE CYCLE

The tick's life cycle occupies 3 years. It is also a three-host tick. All stages of development – larva, nymph and adult – feed on the host for a short time and then return to the ground cover.

DISEASES

Louping ill, tick-borne fever and redwater fever are all transmitted by *Ixodes ricinus*.

LOUPING ILL (AETIOLOGICAL AGENT LOUPING ILL VIRUS)

Distribution

Louping ill is predominantly a disease of sheep but it can occur in cattle. Red grouse may also be affected in the areas where the disease is endemic in the sheep. Ticks appear only to acquire new infection from sheep or grouse and as transovarial transmission does not appear to occur with this disease it would be impossible for it to be sustained by cattle alone.

Louping ill occurs in cattle in the West Highlands, Scottish Borders and in a small area on Bodmin Moor.

Clinical findings

Following an incubation period of 6–18 days there is the onset of a high fever coinciding with the viraemic phase. This subsides and often goes unnoticed and up to 5 days later clinical signs occur heralding the invasion of the central nervous system and are accompanied by the return of fever. The signs are of an encephalomyelitis, shown in Table 19.1.

Treatment

In many cases, particularly in lactating cows, treatment for hypomagnesaemia will have been administered to no effect (apart from those measures aimed at sedation). Cattle should recover over a period of 2 days if kept quiet in a darkened box.

Clinical diagnosis

Diagnosis can cause confusion because of the similarity of the disease to other diseases causing derangement of the central nervous system. Therefore the class of livestock, location, proximity of sheep and time of year are all important initial considerations.

Laboratory diagnosis

Suitable material for laboratory diagnosis is available from animals which have been shot. Histology, particularly of the brain stem, virus isolation from brain and serology are required. Because of the late appearance of clinical signs in the course of the disease, serology is useful at an early stage.

Control

Louping ill vaccine provides good protection and the two-dose programme should be completed at least 2 weeks before exposure to the disease.

Table 19.1 Signs of louping ill.

Hyperaesthesia	Rigidity of gait
Blinking	Circling in some cases
Rolling of the eyes	Convulsions and coma
Muscle tremors	

TICK-BORNE FEVER (AETIOLOGICAL AGENT – *RICKETTSIA CYTOECETES PHAGOCYTOPHILA*)

Tick-borne fever is widespread and occurs wherever *Ixodes ricinus* is found. Though predominantly a sheep disease, it also affects cattle. Unlike louping ill and redwater fever, most ticks are carriers.

Clinical findings

The clinical findings are as follows:

(1)   After an incubation period of 7–10 days there is onset of fever (40.5–41.5°C) [105–107°F] which lasts 3–8 days in untreated cases.
(2)   Cattle become stiff and are reluctant to move; the hock region is often filled.
(3)   There is a loss of appetite.
(4)   Respiratory rate increases and there is occasional coughing and harsh lung sounds.
(5)   Milk yields are depressed.
(6)   Secondary effects such as abortion and respiratory disease are consequent upon white cell depression.

The disease is seldom seen in cattle under 15 months. Untreated animals make a slow recovery but weight loss and reduction in milk yield can be marked and prolonged.

Diagnosis

Diagnosis may be confirmed at the height of the febrile stage by examination of Giemsa-stained smears which show typical tick-borne fever bodies in the eosinophils and neutrophils.

Treatment

Good response is achieved with oxytetracycline and sulphonamide therapy.

Control

As the disease is endemic in the south western peninsula of England its economic importance is not known and one assumes that, as in the case of redwater fever, exposure to the disease early in life confers immunity and only when fully susceptible stock become infected does the full impact of the disease become apparent. Control should therefore be aimed at tick control (see later) by early-in-life exposure of cattle.

REDWATER FEVER (AETIOLOGICAL AGENT, *BABESIA DIVERGENS*

All stages of the tick's development have been shown to transmit *Babesia divergens* but only the adult female may acquire new infection from either a clinically affected or premune carrier host.

Clinical findings

In field cases the period from tick bite to clinical disease is probably 7–14 days, the haemoglobinuria ("redwater") appearing 14–21 days after introduction of susceptible stock to the known infective pasture.

The obvious clinical sign of haemoglobinuria makes diagnosis of this condition relatively simple but because of the progressive nature of the disease and the change in treatment thereby occasioned a full clinical assessment of the animal is always necessary.

Early signs

Early signs of the disease are:

(1) Slight dullness associated with rising temperature to 40.5–41.5°C.
(2) Pulse rate normal.
(3) Diarrhoea with spasm of the anal sphincter resulting in a very narrow bore stream of dung "pipe stem faeces". This

frequently produces lines of faeces on the hind legs and flanks – centred at the tail head.
(4)   Appearance of haemoglobinuria. This first appears after the temperature rise.
(5)   Slight dehydration with hollowing around the eye.
(6)   The pupil is dilated.
(7)   Appetite and thirst normal.

Signs after 24–36 h

(1)   Temperature 39–39.5°C, pulse rising and some pallor of mucous membranes.
(2)   Faeces normal, anal spasm still present.
(3)   Urine dark in colour and reduced in quantity.
(4)   Less willing to move.
(5)   Reduction in appetite and thirst.
(6)   Reduction in milk yield.

After a further 24–36 h

(1)   Temperature subnormal, pulse rate 120 or more. Respiratory rate increased, mucous membranes markedly pale and also jaundiced. Typical of profound haemolytic anaemia.
(2)   Faeces very dry and orange-coloured because of excess bile staining. Animal is very constipated.
(3)   Urine is absent or if present black in colour.
(4)   Animal is frequently recumbent and much embarrassed by any movement. Groaning is an extremely bad sign and probably due to angina.
(5)   Appetite is small or nil and the thirst similar.

The appearance of the urine can given an indication as to the stage of development of the disease and can best be described in vintner's terms from early to late and finally clearing, i.e. rosé, burgundy, claret, port, Guinness, ginger (clearing).

Diagnosis

Diagnosis depends on epidemiological evidence (class of livestock, location and time of year), haemoglobinuria and other clinical signs and examination of Giemsa-stained smears prepared from blood taken at the early, febrile, stage of the disease (Figs 19.3–19.5).

These will reveal the twin widely separated "Indian club"

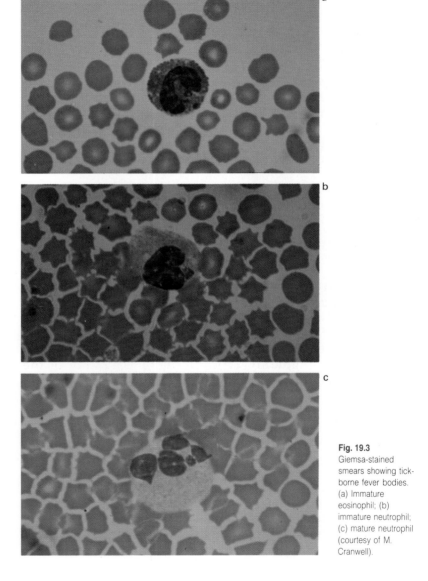

Fig. 19.3
Giemsa-stained smears showing tick-borne fever bodies. (a) Immature eosinophil; (b) immature neutrophil; (c) mature neutrophil (courtesy of M. Cranwell).

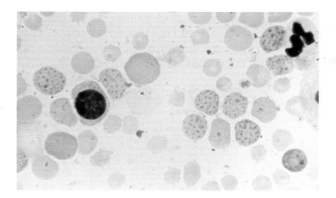

Fig. 19.4
Severe haemolytic
anaemia. Giemsa-
stained smear
showing anisocytosis
(erythrocytes of
different sizes),
polychromasia
(young erythrocytes
taking up more or
less strain according
to amount of
haemoglobin present)
and reticulocytosis
(basophilic stippling)
(Crown copyright).

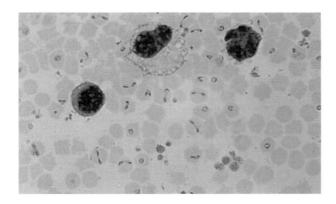

Fig. 19.5
Parasitaemia showing
Babesia divergens
(Giemsa stain)
(Crown copyright).

shaped organisms typically occuring at the periphery of the
erythrocyte. *Babesia divergens* is, however, pleomorphic and
other shapes are commonly encountered.

Treatment

Cases treated in the early stages of the disease normally
respond very quickly to a subcutaneous injection of imidocarb
dipropionate 12 % w/v (Imizol; Pitman-Moore) given at
1 ml/100 kg. Only one injection is permitted.

Revisits

Owners of cattle fulfilling one or more of the following conditions are advised to request revisits in 24 h:

(1) The urine has not cleared or is not clearing (ginger colour).
(2) There is marked inappetence.
(3) There is marked constipation ("stoppage").
(4) There is marked weakness and prolonged recumbency.

Cases which are first seen at a more advanced stage of the disease will have to receive more initial treatment and frequently result in revisits, often at the instigation of the veterinarian. The revisit rate is 11–12 %.

Treatment

Mineral/vitamin/food supplement appetite stimulants such as Leo Cud (Leo) are employed. Farmers frequently supply ivy and also a pan of earth as redwater cases develop a craving for it, no doubt in an attempt to replace iron. Iron complex injections can be given to do this.

Constipation is traditionally treated with black treacle which provides food as well as being laxative. Liquid paraffin may also be administered. Oral treatments are best administered quietly by stomach tube as any struggling in severely anaemic and dehydrated animals can be fatal.

Dehydration is corrected by administration of parenteral fluids (Isolec; Ivex International).

For those cases whose urine has cleared, which still remain weak and show marked anaemia often accompanied by jaundice, whole blood transfusion can be life saving. With reference to transfusion it has been said:

> Transfusion therapy is basically an attempt to replace blood or its components when life is threatened without such restoration. Undoubtedly it is often a life saving measure but it has the potential of doing as much harm as the condition it is designed to alleviate. While this should not deter the use of transfusion in clinical practice when indicated, transfusion should be instituted with extreme caution and care.

In vitro tests for donor/recipient compatability are unreliable and an *in vivo* test involving the injection of 100–200 ml of blood into the recipient and waiting for 10–30 min for signs of shock to develop is the best plan of action. As transfusion reactions produce haemolysis this reinforces our rule of only transfusing animals in which the haemolytic process has been arrested, i.e. the urine has cleared or is clearing.

The most difficult part of the operation is collection and a donor is selected bearing the following in mind:

(1) Related or the same breed – not essential.
(2) Suffering from no intercurrent disease – check the urine.
(3) Not in advanced pregnancy.
(4) Quiet to handle.

An excellent description of blood transfusion in cattle was given by MacKellar in 1962 and the method employed today, apart from minor modifications, is essentially the same.

In order to exclude any possible reactions caused by airborne particles a closed method of collection is now used. The plastic tube leading from the 5 mm collecting needle is fitted through the giving top of a 5 l collapsible collection bag (Infusor; Combi-set). Proprietory anticoagulant (Anticoagulant; Bimeda) is first placed in the bag and flushed through the collecting needle and tube. Up to 10 l of blood are used and the patient also receives parenteral fluids. Infusion rates of up to 250 ml/min can be used without shock occurring but care must be taken not to embarrass very sick animals by overloading their circulation.

The effects of transfusion are often immediate. Though the blood volume administered is small in terms of total blood volume in a normal animal, when added to the greatly depleted volume of the long-term redwater case its relative effect can be great and recumbent animals will often rise, drink and commence feeding.

Redwater fever can be fatal but, at any of the described stages, the untreated animal may recover spontaneously or finally in spite of treatment at an early stage some animals will die. The death can be due to dehydration, anaemia, toxaemia, shock or a combination of all these factors. Recovered animals are immune and this immunity is retained if it be reinforced.

Age susceptibility

Calves under 6 months old do not become clinically affected
but do acquire premunity.

PRACTICE RECORDS OF REDWATER FEVER CASES

AIR TEMPERATURE EFFECTS

Seasonal incidence of redwater fever has been recorded in
the Tavistock practice since 1956. The typical two peak
characteristic of the disease incidence graph is shown in Fig.
19.6 and represents the seasonal difference in response of the
vector *Ixodes ricinus* to temperature. Analysis of the seasonal
incidence of redwater fever over the years 1955 to 1967 showed
a very significant correlation with maximum air temperature
provided that the periods January to May (spring) and June
to October (autumn) were considered separately. This further
confirmed the existence of two distinct populations of ticks.
The response of spring ticks to rise in temperature was two-
and-a-half times that of the autumn ticks. The same basic
monthly pattern is maintained for 1984–1986 (Fig. 19.7).

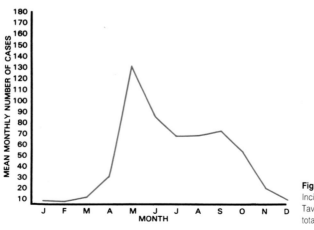

Fig. 19.6
Incidence of redwater in
Tavistock. Mean monthly
totals 1956–1966.

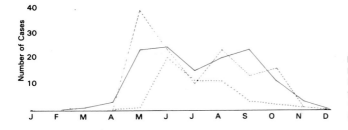

Fig. 19.7
Redwater incidence
in Tavistock. Monthly
totals, 1984 (red);
1985 (blue); 1986
(green).

ANNUAL DIFFERENCES IN INCIDENCE

A final fact emerges in that the difference in annual totals is paralleled and therefore created by the difference in autumn cases (Fig. 19.8). In order to maintain this relationship in 1986 the June case incidence had to be transferred to the spring tick total. Cold temperatures were maintained until June in 1986 and therefore the author feels that this "cheating" is valid.

CONTROL OF THE DISEASE

Control may be directed at the tick and also at the livestock.

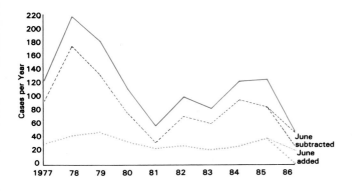

Fig. 19.8
Redwater incidence
in Tavistock. Annual
totals 1977–1987
(red) showing spring
(green) and autumn
(blue) totals.

Tick control

Ticks can be controlled using the following methods:

(1)   Reduce tick cover by good grass husbandry – close grazing, ploughing up or burning old pasture.
(2)   Scavenge tick pastures with sheep. As transovarial transmission occurs this will not remove the reservoir of infection but will dilute the challenge. Ticks present at dipping will be killed.
(3)   Use of spray or pour-on pyrethroids to confer protection.
(4)   Use of pour-on warble treatment in the spring after March 15.

Livestock management

Livestock management is as follows:

(1)   Expose young stock to tick pastures before 6 months and thereby acquire premunity. This is every effective.
(2)   Imidocarb dipropionate (Imizol; Pitman-Moore) can be used subcutaneously at the prophylactic rate of 2.5 ml/100 kg. The whole group is injected either (a) when susceptible stock is introduced to a known redwater pasture, or (b) following the first clinical case. Tissue levels of imidocarb dipropionate are elevated for a considerable time, thus allowing susceptible stock to acquire premunity when *Babesia*-carrying ticks infest them.

The prolonged tissue levels also explain the extremely precise conditions of usage, and no doubt the long period taken for it to be licenced.

PAST AND PRESENT INCIDENCE OF REDWATER

Examination of our recent records from 1977 to 1986 compared with 1956 to 1966 shows a tremendous fall in case numbers of redwater fever (Fig. 19.9). The all-time low of 49 cases occurred in 1986.

To repeat, two factors are necessary for tick-borne disease in cattle – ticks and susceptible livestock.

Factors which could have affected tick numbers

These can be listed as follows:

(1)   Changed grass husbandry. There has been a general swing to silage as opposed to hay – the crop is taken earlier and cut far lower. Further cuts are also taken. The ticks' habitat is opened up and disturbed more.
(2)   Advent of the turbo-mower which produces a far more even and lower cut than the previous finger mower thereby producing a drier environment.
(3)   More sheep are kept and compulsory dipping has returned – now with organophosphorous compounds.
(4)   Organophosphorus and pyrethroid ear tags have been introduced for cattle for fly control.
(5)   Compulsory warble treatment has taken place.
(6)   Ivermectin has been introduced.
(7)   Springs "seem" colder and later in onset.

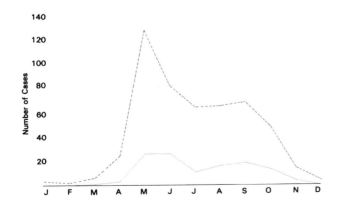

Fig. 19.9
Redwater incidence in Tavistock. Mean monthly totals 1956–1966 (red) and 1976–1986 (green).

Factors affecting cattle susceptibility

Most cattle in the Tavistock area are now home bred. There are few of the butcher/graziers who used to buy in highly susceptible forward stores to finish on the permanent tick pastures.

Such a dramatic fall in disease incidence is worthy of explanation and hopefully an investigation of the known tick pastures will furnish the answer to the question "is *Ixodes ricinus* a dying breed?"

ACKNOWLEDGEMENT

For the section of this article devoted to redwater I am indebted to the original work initiated on this disease by my late partner J. C. MacKellar FRCVS. In this work he was greatly assisted by J. Donnelly.

REFERENCES AND FURTHER READING

Cranwell, M. P. & Gibbons, J. A. (1986). *Veterinary Record* **119**, 531–532.
Donnelly, J. & MacKellar, J. C. (1970). *Agricultural Meteorology* **7**, 5–17.
Donnelly, J. & Pierce, M. A. (1975). *International Journal for Parasitology* **74**, 363–367.
MacKellar, J. C. (1962). *Veterinary Record* **74**, 763–765.
Reid, H. W. (1987). *In Practice* **9**, 189.
Wilson, J. C., Foggie, A. & Carmichael, M. A. (1964). *Veterinary Record* **76**, 1081.

CHAPTER 20

Prevention of Calf Diarrhoea by Vaccination

DAVID SNODGRASS

INTRODUCTION

Much progress has been made over recent years in unravelling the complex aetiology of calf scour. Surveys throughout the UK suggest that, although many infectious agents have the potential to cause diarrhoea in calves, there is a limited number that commonly do so. Rotavirus infection is the most frequently diagnosed under all systems of calf husbandry. Infections with *Cryptosporidium* species, *Salmonella* species (particularly in calves purchased through markets), coronavirus and enterotoxigenic *Escherichia coli* are also of significance.

Of these agents, the two that lend themselves most readily to vaccine development are rotavirus and enterotoxigenic *E. coli*. Immunity to cryptosporidial infection is not well understood, and *in vitro* cultivation of the parasite is not easily achieved. With coronavirus there have been problems in obtaining adequate virus titres for vaccines from cell culture. Development and improvement of *Salmonella* species vaccines is a subject that requires separate consideration.

IMMUNIZATION

The two approaches possible for preventing infectious disease in young animals are either by active immunization of the newborn or, by passive immunization through dam vaccination. A modified-live rotavirus vaccine was developed over a decade ago in the USA for oral administration to calves on the day of birth. However, there is evidence that this vaccine is ineffective in the field, probably because of near-simultaneous ingestion of colostrum containing antibody to rotavirus which neutralized the vaccine virus. The major emphasis in vaccine development has therefore been put on dam vaccination, although it is possible that live rotavirus vaccines may have a role in the future in actively immunizing calves brought on to farms at a few days of age.

The passive immunization problems presented by rotavirus and enterotoxigenic *E. coli* are different. Rotavirus is probably endemic in all herds and hence all cows produce antibody to rotavirus in colostrum for the first 3–4 days after calving, although not subsequently in milk. This antibody, ingested by all colostrum-fed calves, is the principal protective mechanism against clinical rotavirus diarrhoea and, at the least, is usually effective at delaying rotavirus diarrhoea problems until the calf is 4–5 days of age. The important principle underlying protection is that antibody present in the lumen of the gut, and not that absorbed into the circulation, is the most effective at preventing rotavirus diarrhoea. Therefore, with rotavirus vaccines the aim is not only to increase colostral antibody titres but also to prolong antibody secretion in post-colostral milk.

ENTEROTOXIGENIC *E. COLI*

Enterotoxigenic *E. coli* are not endemic in the UK and only about 3 % of cows possess antibody. Disease occurs sporadically and presents as an acute watery diarrhoea in very young calves, usually 1–2 days of age. As a result of this age restriction, colostral antibody alone is sufficient to protect calves. Although enterotoxigenic *E. coli* belong to several different O and K serogroups, they share common virulence determinants in the fimbrial adhesin known as K99 and in the heat-stable toxin ST. The toxin is poorly antigenic, but K99 provides a readily available source of antigen for vaccine formulation. A K99-based enterotoxigenic *E. coli* vaccine is already available in the UK.

ROTAVIRUS VACCINES

The use of a good adjuvant is important for rotavirus vaccines. Non-adjuvanted rotavirus vaccines available in the USA are largely ineffective, while aluminium hydroxide-adjuvanted rotavirus vaccines have been disappointing experimentally.

In Britain, vaccine has been developed using an inactivated bovine rotavirus with K99 from enterotoxigenic *E. coli*, blended in an oil adjuvant. This vaccine is administered to pregnant cows in a 1.0 ml dose intramuscularly, from 1 to 3 months before calving. In beef suckler herds, vaccination is recommended 1 month before the calving season, with revaccination 3 months later for any uncalved cows. In dairy herds, vaccination at drying off is a simple and effective routine.

No alteration of management to ensure continued ingestion of antibody is necessary in beef suckler herds. However, in dairy herds it is essential that calves are fed from colostrum pools for the first 2 weeks of life. These pools from the first 4 days' milkings from several cows will be of more uniform antibody titre than the declining quality available from the dam alone. They may be stored at ambient temperature for a few days without loss of efficacy, or they may be stored frozen.

Field trials in the UK of a rotavirus/K99 vaccine have shown protection against rotavirus infection and diarrhoea in both beef and suckler herds. Experimental challenge with enterotoxigenic *E. coli* showed excellent protection against the K99 component of the vaccine.

A vaccine based on these principles is now available in the UK as a prescription only medicine. It should prove of considerable benefit in controlling calf scour caused by rotavirus and enterotoxigenic *E. coli*, particularly when used in combination with good management practices. Its availability will put an onus on practitioners and diagnostic laboratories to provide an accurate and rapid differential diagnosis of the several agents potentially involved in scour problems. Appropriate laboratory diagnostic techniques are now available. It will also provide an opportunity for veterinary surgeons to add specific prophylaxis to their armament for controlling one of the most perennial and intractable of cattle diseases.

FURTHER READING

Reynolds, D. J., Morgan, J. H., Chanter, N., Jones, P. W., Bridger, J. C., Debney, T. J. & Brach, K. J. (1986). *Veterinary Record* **119**, 34.
Snodgrass, D. R. (1986). *Veterinary Record* **119**, 39.
Snodgrass, D. R., Terzolo, H. R., Sherwood, D., Campbell, I., Menzies, J. D. & Synge, B. A. (1986). *Veterinary Record* **119**, 31.

Index